Demand and need for dental care

A SOCIO–DENTAL STUDY

A report of research undertaken by

J. S. BULMAN, B.D.S.
N. D. RICHARDS, M.A.
G. L. SLACK, O.B.E., T.D., F.D.S., DIP. BACT.
A. J. WILLCOCKS, B.COM., PH.D.

Published for the Nuffield Provincial Hospitals Trust
by the Oxford University Press 1968
London New York Toronto

Oxford University Press, Ely House, London W 1
GLASGOW NEW YORK TORONTO MELBOURNE WELLINGTON
CAPE TOWN SALISBURY IBADAN NAIROBI LUSAKA ADDIS ABABA
BOMBAY CALCUTTA MADRAS KARACHI LAHORE DACCA
KUALA LUMPUR HONG KONG TOKYO

Designed by Bernard Crossland
Printed in Great Britain by Alden & Mowbray Ltd
at the Alden Press, Oxford
Bound by the Kemp Hall Bindery, Oxford

Demand and need for dental care

Foreword

This report has been prepared from a fuller report made to the Nuffield Provincial Hospitals Trust. The study reported represents a joint and co-ordinated effort on the part of specialists from two widely contrasting disciplines. It was decided in both instances that the reports would best be prepared and edited by one of us. We must therefore place on record our thanks to N. David Richards who produced the full report and to John S. Bulman for this report. Mr. Richards and Dr. Arthur J. Willcocks (of the applied Social Science Department of the University of Nottingham) have been responsible for the sociological data; Professor Geoffrey L. Slack and Mr. Bulman for the dental data associated with the study.

Although each report was written and edited primarily by one of us (N. D. R. and J. S. B.) this report, as in the first, details the collective endeavours of two social scientists and two dental scientists, and we offer it to the reader, with due apologies for an admitted emphasis on the sociological aspects, as our joint effort. We have been conscious that we have been writing to interest and stimulate, not only the social and dental scientist, but also the layman; for this reason we have therefore been deliberately less specific and more general than we might perhaps otherwise have been. The subject of dental care has hitherto received but scanty attention—there is therefore the need to encourage the layman to take a further and more positive interest in dental health.

Many individuals have contributed in one way or another to the production of this report and the investigations it describes. We cannot name all of them, but we do indeed acknowledge their help.

Certain individuals and bodies must, however, be named—in particular we record our thanks to the Nuffield Provincial Hospitals Trust (and their secretary Mr. G. McLachlan) who made the study possible, and to the Council of Governors of the London Hospital Medical College who provided accommodation and a base for our research unit. We are also grateful to our sociological and dental colleagues in London and Nottingham (particularly to Professor David C. Marsh for kindly allowing us access to the statistical facilities of the Department of Applied Social Science of the University of Nottingham), and also to many persons in the dental services. We have received much helpful assistance from the staff and officials of the General Dental Council, British Dental Association, Federation Dentaire Internationale, Ministry of Health, Dental Estimates Board, and local health authorities and health executive councils in Salisbury and Wiltshire, and in Darlington.

We are indebted to Sir Wilfred Fish, formerly President of the General Dental Council, and to Professor C. A. Moser and his colleagues at L.S.E., who were responsible for developments which led to the undertaking of the studies we report. We also wish to thank Dr. P. W. R. Morpurgo who was intimately concerned with the formulation and early stages of our study, and acted at this time as co-director with Professor G. L. Slack.

We also owe an especial debt to our local staff and in particular to the resourceful and responsible assistance received from our small team of interviewers. Our thanks are also due to many people who in all probability will never see this publication—namely those who so willingly received us into their homes. To all those persons we willingly accord our thanks and gratitude.

Contents

IV. DISCUSSION

APPENDICES

I Introduction

The investigations described in this report originated as the result of a memorandum submitted to the Nuffield Provincial Hospitals Trust by Sir Wilfred Fish, then President of the General Dental Council as well as a member of the Trust's Dental Advisory Group. This memorandum proposed the establishment of a commission to investigate problems concerning dental health and the dental services in this country. Accordingly the Trust invited Professor C. A. Moser and two colleagues from the London School of Economics to review the available facts concerning dental health and services, and their report was published by the Trust in 1962. This report drew attention to a number of deficiencies in the available dental statistics. For example, little was known of the prevalence and distribution of dental disease in the country, or of the difference between the need and the demand for dental treatment, or indeed of the attitude of the general public towards dental health and oral care. The report proposed an investigation into the individual's reaction to all aspects of dental health and the dental services to be carried out in one or possibly more localities. This proposition was accepted by the Trust, who in 1962 provided funds for the establishment at the London Hospital Medical College of a research unit under the direction of Professor G. L. Slack. His terms of reference were, broadly, to obtain from a pilot investigation as much information as possible on community dental health and the individual's attitude towards dental health and the dental services by means of both sociological and dental investigations.

Two contrasting urban areas were chosen for the study, one in the North of England and one in the South; the northern area having a higher than average dentist/population ratio and the southern area having a lower than average dentist/population ratio.

Two approaches were decided upon in conducting the investigation. In the first instance, sociological interviewers would contact every member of a random sample of the survey area population and request their co-operation in completing a detailed questionnaire covering all relevant aspects of the study. At the end of this interview, subjects would be asked if they would be willing to submit to a very brief dental examination. Those who agreed would then be visited at a later date by the survey team's dental surgeon (J. S. B.) who would make a short but detailed assessment of their oral health.

This basic plan was put into operation in 1963 with little modification following a pilot survey in the Hornchurch and Upminster area of Essex to test both the questionnaire and examination techniques to be used.

Survey areas

The two areas chosen were Salisbury with Wilton in Wiltshire, where the number of resident dentists was comparatively high, and Darlington in County Durham where relatively few dentists were available. Both areas had water fluoride levels below the national average.

In choosing suitable areas, it was necessary to find communities which, while large enough to yield useful and significant data, were yet sufficiently self-contained to ensure that the majority of the inhabitants spent their time within the area limits and tended not to travel further afield to obtain dental treatment. For this reason any town within 20 miles or so of a large city was ruled out, as commuters to the city might well attend dentists there and so confuse any data obtained on dental visiting habits. Even so, it was found that in the areas finally chosen some people did travel several miles to obtain dental treatment, but their number was far less than would have been the case in a commuting area.

The Dental Register for 1925 listed 13 dentists as living in

Salisbury and 21 in Darlington. By 1931 the number living in Darlington had increased to 27, while the number in Salisbury had remained constant. At the time of this survey, there were 30 dentists living in Salisbury and 28 in Darlington. It must be remembered, however, that residence does not necessarily imply the general practice of dentistry. Some of the registered dentists had retired, and others were employed in hospital or school dental services. A better idea of the number of dentists available to give routine dental treatment was provided by the local executive councils, which listed 17 dentists working in the General Dental Services of the N.H.S. in both Salisbury and Darlington at the time of the survey. Since the estimated population of the two areas at that time was 39,500 (Salisbury) and 84,200 (Darlington), the dentist/population ratios were 1:2,320 (Salisbury) and 1:4,950 (Darlington). These figures do not include those dentists practising outside the N.H.S. The national dentist/population ratio at this time was 1:4,450, there being 9,991 dentists in the N.H.S. in England and Wales to treat a population of 44,471,757. This ratio was subject to very wide variation throughout the country as the following county table shows:

	County	Dentist/population ratio
South	London	1:2360
	Middlesex	1:2940
	Sussex	1:3020
North Midlands	Staffordshire	1:7480
	Nottinghamshire	1:7283
North	Durham	1:7060
	Cumberland	1:6290

A very brief description of the two areas may help the reader to build up a picture of the communities chosen for this investigation.

Salisbury is essentially a market town and shopping centre with a high proportion of its population employed in the retail and distributive trades. It is the only major shopping centre between Yeovil in the west, Winchester in the east, Bournemouth and Southampton in the south, and Trowbridge and Bath in the north. The extensive use of Salisbury Plain by the Army and Royal Air Force has also influenced the city as a service centre, as does the fact that it lies on main road and rail connections between London and Bristol, Exeter, Bournemouth, and Southampton. There is some local light industry, the Wilton carpet factory being probably the most famous example.

Darlington was for 100 years a railway town, and heavy industry is still there in abundance, but it too is a busy shopping and service centre. It lies on main rail and road connections between London, Newcastle, and Edinburgh.

The sample population

In order to obtain a suitable sample of the populations under investigation the names of 558 adults in Salisbury, and 598 in Darlington were drawn at random from the electoral registers of the two areas. These numbers meant that the sample included 1 adult out of every 50 living in Salisbury and 1 out of every 97 living in Darlington. Of these, 465 in Salisbury and 516 in Darlington were contacted, the remaining 12 per cent (Salisbury), 10 per cent (Darlington) having either died or moved, were too old or too ill to be seen, or could never be found at home. Of those approached, 95 per cent (Salisbury), 96 per cent (Darlington) agreed to be interviewed. As was to be expected, the thought of a dental examination deterred more people than the thought of an interview. Of those interviewed, 82 per cent (Salisbury), 91 per cent (Darlington) agreed at the time to be examined, but second thoughts away from the persuasive influence of the interviewer later reduced these figures to 76 per cent (Salisbury), 86 per cent (Darlington). A further 8 per cent (Salisbury), 7 per cent (Darlington) evaded the net thrown by the dental examiner, so that eventually 68 per cent (Salisbury), 79 per cent (Darlington) of those interviewed were dentally examined. This represented 56 per cent (Salisbury), 68 per cent (Darlington), of the original sample, and was considered to be reasonably satisfactory in view of the novelty of the proposition and the inevitable invasion of privacy involved.

Age-group	Males		Females		Total		Percentage of total		Census data, percentage of population	
21–5	13[1]	20[1]	28	20	41	40	9	8	9	9
26–30	13	22	15	22	28	44	6	9	8	8
31–5	20	14	21	29	41	43	9	8	9	9
36–40	27	19	25	33	52	52	11	10	9	10
41–5	21	30	24	29	45	59	10	11	10	10
46–50	20	26	29	27	49	53	11	11	9	10
51–5	17	27	25	28	42	55	9	11	10	10
56–60	25	20	20	26	45	46	10	9	9	9
61–5	21	14	18	24	39	38	8	7	8	8
66–70	8	12	18	17	26	29	6	6	6	6
Over 70	23	30	34	25	57	55	12	11	13	11
All ages	208	236	257	280	465	516	100	100	100	100

(N.B. The Census Data are presented for slightly different age-groups, viz. 20–4, 25–9, etc.)

1. Roman figures represent Salisbury and italic figures Darlington.

TABLE I.I. *Ages of those interviewed and of those in the population of the two towns. Sample data*

Two major questions now remained to be answered. Did the drawn sample accurately reflect all possible social categories of the two populations, and what bias, if any, was introduced as the result of the reduced numbers interviewed and examined? To find an answer to the first question, the sample figures were compared with the 1961 Census figures and found to correspond closely in sex, age-distribution (five-year groupings), marital status, and in Darlington in socio-economic groupings using the Registrar-General's occupational classifications described in the 1961 Census. In Salisbury the middle social strata were slightly over-represented, with a corresponding under-representation of the two social extremes. This was not enough, however, to affect the representative validity of the sample. The figures of those who were interviewed also compared well with the Census returns. As was to be expected, the examination figures were biased. In both Salisbury and Darlington, women, the elderly, and widows were under-represented, and those who said that they received private dental treatment or who had not been to a dentist for ten years. In Salisbury too the two extremes of the social scale were under-

Social class	Males		Females		Total		Percentage of total	
I	7[1]	*4[1]*	8	*3*	15	*7*	3	*1*
II	32	*12*	41	*30*	73	*42*	16	*8*
III non-manual	29	*35*	64	*56*	93	*91*	20	*18*
III manual	102	*121*	103	*127*	205	*248*	44	*48*
IV	25	*39*	28	*40*	53	*79*	11	*15*
V	12	*24*	10	*22*	25	*46*	5	*9*
Unknown	1	*1*	3	*2*	4	*3*	1	*1*
All classes	208	*236*	257	*280*	465	*516*	100	*100*

1. Roman figures represent Salisbury and italic figures Darlington.

TABLE I.2. *The social class distribution of those interviewed*

represented. This is of some significance as apart from the small number of private patients and younger women involved, these categories would have produced a high incidence of poor dental health or full dentures; information lost to the data on dental health given in Part II of this Report. In other words the picture of dental health painted in Part II is a little brighter than was actually the case.

The social status of the sample was determined on an occupational basis using the Registrar-General's classification of occupations. This makes use of five classes, the third of which was further subdivided for more detailed analysis in the survey:

Class I. 'Professional' occupations
    II. 'Intermediate' occupations   } 'NON-MANUAL'
    III. Non-manual } 'Skilled' occupations
    III. Manual
    IV. 'Semi-skilled' occupations   } 'MANUAL'
    V. 'Unskilled' occupations

In the case of women, the husband's occupation or former occupation was used.

This classification showed up some significant differences between the two areas. Sixty-one per cent of the Salisbury sample interviewed were manual workers, ex-manual workers, or the wives of manual workers and 39 per cent were non-manual workers (Classes I, II, and III non-manual). In Darlington only

	Males	Females	Total	Percentage of total
Single	15[1] *34*[1]	47 *31*	62 *65*	13 *13*
Married	177 *183*	167 *205*	344 *388*	74 *75*
Widowed	11 *19*	38 *41*	49 *60*	11 *12*
Divorced	5 —	5 *3*	10 *3*	2 *1*
All groups	208 *236*	257 *280*	465 *516*	100 *100*

1. Roman figures represent Salisbury and italic figures Darlington.

TABLE I.3. *Marital status of those interviewed*

27 per cent were non-manual workers. In both towns Class III contained 65 per cent of the total sample interviewed, 45 per cent manual and 20 per cent non-manual in Salisbury, and 47 per cent manual, 18 per cent non-manual in Darlington. Because of the lack of numbers in Class I, Classes I and II were combined and together contained 19 per cent of the Salisbury total and 9 per cent of the Darlington total. Classes IV and V contained 16 per cent of the Salisbury total and 24 per cent of the Darlington total. In Darlington 82 per cent, and in Salisbury 85 per cent, of the men interviewed were working, 14 per cent in Salisbury and 17 per cent in Darlington had retired and 1 per cent were unemployed. There were more working women in Salisbury, 24 per cent of the Salisbury women interviewed being in full-time occupation and 17 per cent working part-time compared to 20 and 12 per cent respectively in Darlington. Marital state figures were the same in both towns, 75 per cent of those interviewed being married, 13

	Number		Percentage	
Males				
Working	177[1]	*193*[1]	38	*37*
Not working/unemployed	2	*3*	—	*1*
Retired	29	*40*	6	*8*
Females				
Working full-time	63	*57*	14	*11*
Working part-time	43	*33*	9	*6*
Not working	151	*190*	32	*37*
All groups	465	*516*	100	*100*

1. Roman figures represent Salisbury and italic figures Darlington.

TABLE I.4. *Occupational status of those interviewed*

per cent single, 11 per cent widowed, and 1–2 per cent divorced. Age figures were also similar, in both towns 45 per cent of the sample interviewed were over 50 and 84–6 per cent over 30.

This sample population represented all adults over the age of 21, but included no younger people. It was therefore decided also to interview any young people between the ages of 15 and 21 met within the families of the main sample. No claim is made that this was a fully representative sample of 'teenagers' in the areas, but it fell not too far short of the ideal. One hundred and twenty-eight of these 'teenagers' were listed in Salisbury and 147 in Darlington, and of these 116 (91 per cent) were interviewed in Salisbury and 133 (90 per cent) in Darlington. One hundred and one (79 per cent) were examined in Salisbury and 115 (78 per cent) in Darlington.

A record was kept of the composition of all families visited including the ages and sex of all children. Wherever possible, all willing members of a 'sample' family were examined at the same time as the main subject although to avoid complicating this report these ancillary data have not been included. The youngest person examined was just over 1 year old and the oldest over 90. To obtain more dental information on children under 15 years of

S.E.G.		Number		Percentage	
1 and 2	Employers and managers	48[1]	28[1]	10	5
3 and 4	Professional	15	7	3	1
5 and 6	Intermediate and Junior, non-manual	112	108	24	21
7	Personal service	11	6	2	1
8	Foremen and supervisors, manual	15	32	3	6
9	Skilled manual	171	209	37	41
10	Semi-skilled manual	39	70	8	14
11	Unskilled manual	22	45	5	9
12	Own accord workers (not professional)	19	2	4	—
13 and 14	Farmers	2	3	—	1
15	Agricultural workers	7	3	2	1
16	Armed forces	2	—	—	—
17	Indefinite (imprecise data)	2	3	—	1
	All socio-economic groups	465	516	100	100

1. Roman figures represent Salisbury and italic figures Darlington.

TABLE 1.5. *Socio-economic groupings (S.E.G.) of those interviewed*

S.E.G. Groups	Census		Survey	
A. 1, 2, 3, 4, and 13	13[1]	*11*[1]	14	*7*
B. 5, 6, 8, 9, 12, and 14	59	*63*	68	*68*
C. 7, 10, 11, 15, 16, and 17	28	*26*	18	*25*
All groups	100	*100*	100	*100*

1. Roman figures represent Salisbury and italic figures Darlington.

TABLE 1.6. *Comparison of socio-economic grouping (in percentages) between survey data and census data*

age in the areas, examinations of schoolchildren at two infant and two secondary modern schools in Salisbury and one infant and two secondary modern schools in Darlington, were carried out with the generous permission and co-operation of the authorities concerned. In this way 1,045 children were examined in Salisbury and 560 in Darlington. While in no way representative of all the children of the area, these examinations provided valuable comparative information on dental health differences between the two areas in this age-range. (See Appendix C.)

The Interviews

A copy of the questionnaire used in the Survey is included as an appendix to this Report. (Appendix A.)

Interviews were mainly carried out by three or more locally recruited interviewers with experience of this type of work. In each area some interviews were also undertaken by one of the authors (N. D. R.) to keep a check on typical local responses. The pilot study had shown that care needed to be taken to avoid ambiguous or confusing questions; for example, a question on crown and bridge work had to be dropped after the discovery that the average person had no idea what a dental crown or bridge was!

Interviewers were asked to make three attempts to contact the subjects allocated to them, preferably at different times of the day. If all three attempts failed, a different interviewer was sent for one final attempt after which the subject was recorded as a 'non-contact'. Interviewing and examining took approximately six

B

months in each area, Salisbury being visited first between April and September 1963 and Darlington between September 1963 and March 1964.

	Numbers		A		Percentage in groups B		C	
Total interviewed	465[1]	516[1]	68	79	14	12	18	9
Sex								
Males	208	236	77	86	13	4	10	10
Females	257	280	60	74	15	13	25	14
Age-group								
21–5	41	40	90	85	5	10	5	5
26–30	28	44	82	89	18	9	—	2
31–5	41	43	85	81	5	9	10	9
36–40	52	52	73	69	15	21	12	10
41–5	45	59	69	83	22	12	9	5
46–50	49	55	71	85	12	11	16	4
51–5	42	55	55	91	26	4	19	5
56–60	45	46	56	78	16	15	28	7
61–5	39	38	77	74	5	13	18	13
66–70	26	29	46	76	12	14	42	10
Over 70	57	55	46	60	19	15	35	23
Social class								
I and II	88	49	64	82	16	14	20	4
III non-manual	93	91	76	78	11	8	13	14
III manual	205	248	69	78	14	14	17	8
IV	53	79	66	82	17	11	17	6
V	25	46	50	85	23	7	27	9
Indefinite	4	—	—	—	—	—	—	—
Marital status								
Single	62	65	56	69	26	14	18	17
Married	344	388	74	82	12	12	15	5
Widowed	49	60	51	68	12	12	37	20
Divorced } Separated }	10	3	30	—	50	—	20	—

Key: Group A = Originally agreed to dental examination and were subsequently examined.

Group B = Originally agreed to dental examination but were not subsequently examined.

Group C = Refused dental examination when interviewed.

1. Roman figures represent Salisbury and italic figures Darlington.

TABLE 1.7. *Analysis of subjects who were dentally examined and of those who were not examined*

The Examinations

The examination team was provided with a small two-wheeled examination trailer towed by a Land Rover. Examinations could therefore be carried out either in this trailer or in a respondents own home, whichever he or she preferred. In practice the trailer was used more in Salisbury and home visits were more common in Darlington. The dental team consisted of one of the authors (J. S. B.) who acted as sole dental examiner, a secretary to record information obtained, and a locally recruited driver.

The dental examination, which lasted for about three minutes per person, covered dental, periodontal, dento-facial, and prosthetic aspects of oral health. Decayed, missing, and filled teeth and tooth surfaces were noted together with the types of restoration used. Periodontal disease was judged by the degrees of gum inflammation and pocketing present, and details of all dentures worn were noted. Gross orthodontic abnormalities were noted together with other dento-facial anomalies such as cleft lip or cleft palate, but minor orthodontic irregularities were not included.

Illumination for the examinations was provided in the trailer by a 12-volt 'Miralux' dental lamp and in homes by a 4½-volt 'Klinostik' head lamp. Examination aids included a dental mirror, disposable dental probes, a periodontal probe to assess gum pocket depth, and a chip syringe to clean tooth surfaces. No attempt was made to assess oral cleanliness, but calculus deposition was recorded.

No-one who was examined objected to the examination procedure and many who came expecting to experience some discomfort were agreeably surprised. Several 'examination refusals' were converted to acceptances after seeing a friend or relative emerge unscathed from the ordeal. The most common reactions were 'I don't see how I can help—I only have dentures' from older people, and 'I expect my teeth are in a terrible state but please don't tell me as I'd rather not know' from young people. Both parties were reassured to the best of our ability and all information was recorded in a simple code so that the volunteer learned little from what was said. For ethical reasons no opinion was given on the state of any individual's oral health and any questions to the examiner touching on any such matter were invariably met with a suggestion that the subject's own dentist was the only person qualified to deal with the query. All volunteers were assured that their anonymity would be respected.

Introduction to dental data

Part II of this Report presents data on the actual oral state of the samples examined in Salisbury and Darlington, as it appeared to a visiting dental surgeon. Probably no two dentists would ever entirely agree on suitable criteria for an assessment of this nature, but the dental examiner followed as closely as possible the recommendations of the World Health Organization for surveys of this nature,[1] checking his consistency both by repeating examinations throughout the duration of the investigation and by carrying out check examinations with the Director both before, during, and after the survey. The result of these checks was that there was no appreciable variation in the examiner's standards throughout the year in which examinations were conducted.

Combining the various aspects of oral health—dental decay, periodontal disease, missing teeth, or denture status—into one index of oral health has not yet been satisfactorily accomplished. The method used in this Report and briefly outlined in Appendix D merely demonstrates the concept since among other faults it provides no information at all on treatment needs. It does, however, give a useful basis for comparing actual oral health with a subject's own assessment and for this reason data provided by this oral health grading are included at the end of Part II which now follows. All data in this section refer to the adult sample only.

1. W.H.O. Technical Publication 242.

II

Dental data

Missing teeth

The maximum number of teeth a person can possess is 32, but in many people the 'wisdom' teeth never properly appear and so a perfectly sound dentition may be made up of only 28 or 30 teeth. In Salisbury only 9 per cent of the sample examined had 28 or more standing teeth, and in Darlington only 6 per cent; all persons in this category in both towns being under 45 years of age. In Salisbury 42 per cent had no teeth at all, the figure for Darlington being 51 per cent. Salisbury adults averaged 12 teeth per person and Darlington adults 10 teeth per person. Teeth seemed to be lost on average at the rate of one every two years from the age of 21 onwards. In fact most people of 45 or over had full dentures in Darlington although in Salisbury the age was 55 and over.

Age-group	Males		Females		All persons	
21–30	24[1]	*24*[1]	23	*22*	23	*23*
31–40	19	*17*	16	*17*	18	*17*
41–50	13	*11*	11	*4*	12	*8*
51–60	7	*4*	6	*1*	6	*3*
61–70	3	*2*	1	*5*	2	*4*
Over 70	—	*—*	—	*1*	—	*1*

Average number of teeth per person
   Salisbury: 12 present, 18 missing
   Darlington: 10 present, 20 missing

   1. Roman figures represent Salisbury and italic figures Darlington.

TABLE II.I. *Average numbers of standing teeth*

TABLE II.2. Dentition—Numbers of teeth present

Number of teeth present	Sex Males	Females	Age-groups 21-5	26-30	31-5	36-40	41-5	46-50	51-5	56-60	61-5	66-70	Over 70	Social class I and II	III non-manual	III manual	IV and V	All groups
SALISBURY																		
Number	160	155	37	23	35	38	31	35	23	25	30	12	26	56	71	142	46	315
Percentages																		
28 or more	8	9	30	17	14	11	13	—	—	—	—	—	—	16	10	7	4	9
24 or more	27	27	79	56	48	29	36	11	4	—	3	—	—	36	34	22	24	28
20 or more	39	35	87	65	68	47	46	25	17	4	3	—	—	57	44	29	28	38
16 or more	48	47	90	87	82	58	59	33	43	16	6	—	—	67	55	40	35	48
12 or more	52	53	92	100	82	74	62	36	52	16	9	8	—	69	61	45	43	53
8 or more	55	56	92	100	85	76	68	44	52	20	12	8	—	71	64	49	43	56
4 or more	56	57	92	100	80	76	68	44	52	20	17	8	—	71	64	51	43	57
Some	58	59	92	100	89	76	68	51	57	20	17	17	8	71	66	54	43	58
None	42	41	8	—	11	24	32	49	43	80	83	83	92	29	34	46	57	42
	100	100	100	100	100	100	100	100	100	100	100	100	100	100	100	100	100	100
DARLINGTON																		
Number	202	207	34	39	35	36	49	47	50	36	28	22	33	40	71	193	104	409[1]
Percentages																		
28 or more	6	6	32	21	9	6	4	—	—	—	—	—	—	20	11	4	2	6
24 or more	18	19	67	52	40	31	10	9	—	—	—	—	—	35	22	19	10	18
20 or more	32	34	85	83	63	59	22	22	8	3	7	23	—	48	43	32	22	33
16 or more	40	38	94	88	66	70	26	34	16	6	7	27	—	53	49	37	30	39
12 or more	41	41	97	90	72	73	32	38	18	6	7	27	6	58	52	39	31	41
8 or more	45	45	97	92	83	75	40	36	20	12	11	27	6	64	56	46	38	45
4 or more	48	46	100	92	86	75	46	36	22	17	11	27	12	64	56	46	38	47
Some	50	47	100	92	86	75	46	36	22	17	18	27	12	67	56	47	38	49
None	50	53	—	8	14	25	54	64	78	83	82	73	88	33	44	53	62	51
	100	100	100	100	100	100	100	100	100	100	100	100	100	100	100	100	100	100

1. Because of imprecise occupational data one person could not be classified by social class.

Tooth loss was found to be related to social status in spite of the fact that young people were slightly over-represented in the non-manual classes and older people over-represented in the manual classes. In Salisbury, for example, only 28 per cent of Classes I and II were edentulous—that is, they had no teeth left—compared with 56 per cent in Classes IV and V. The figures for Darlington were 33 and 61 per cent.

Women tended to lose teeth earlier than men. In almost every 10-year age-range from 21 onwards the average woman had fewer teeth than the average man.

Untreated dental decay

Since the number of teeth a person has may vary between 0 and 32, to report dental decay in terms of the number of decayed teeth present would be meaningless. Therefore data presented here refer to the proportion of decayed and untreated teeth in the mouth. Wearers of full upper and lower dentures are not included.

Approximately one-quarter of those subjects with teeth of their own were free from untreated dental decay, slightly fewer in Darlington than in Salisbury. Two-thirds had active decay in up to one-third of their teeth, slightly more in Darlington than in Salisbury. One in ten in both towns had more than one-third of their teeth decayed. Assuming therefore that the samples accurately reflected the populations of the two areas, it follows that there were in Salisbury over 11,000, and in Darlington 20,000, persons over the age of 21 needing dental treatment for decay alone. These figures do not include children and teenagers, in whom dental decay is even more extensive.

Women tended to have fewer untreated decayed teeth than men, the difference being greater in Darlington, where 26 per cent of women had no decay compared with 18 per cent of men, than in Salisbury where 30 per cent of the women were free from decay compared with 26 per cent of the men.

Age did not seem to affect the untreated decay pattern in either town except in the under-30s, where the proportion with more than a third of their teeth decayed was considerably higher than

	Males		Females		All persons	
Number	160[1]	*202*[1]	155	*207*	315	*409*
Percentages						
Subject has:						
No teeth present	43	*50*	41	*53*	42	*51*
No decayed teeth present	15	*9*	17	*12*	16	*11*
Up to one-third decayed	36	*37*	38	*30*	37	*33*
Over one-third and up to two-thirds decayed	6	*4*	3	*4*	4	*4*
Over two-thirds decayed	1	*—*	1	*—*	1	*—*
	100	*100*	100	*100*	100	*100*

1. Roman figures represent Salisbury and italic figures Darlington.

TABLE II.3. *Decayed teeth*

the average, with a lowering of the 'nil or less than a third' proportion. This was to be expected as this age-group possessed more teeth than the average, especially posterior decay-prone teeth which in older people had either been lost as a result of decay or periodontal disease or else been restored.

Manual workers had more untreated decayed teeth than non-manual workers. In Salisbury 40 per cent of Classes I and II were free from untreated decay compared with 15 per cent in Classes IV and V, with Darlington producing similar figures.

Restored teeth

Data are again presented in terms of the proportion of teeth restored by fillings, crowns, and bridges, and for this presentation full-denture wearers have again been excluded.

The presence of restored teeth shows that the subject has at some time in his life received conservative dental treatment as opposed to extractions. Probably many people with no restored teeth present at the time of our examination may have had teeth restored once but subsequent neglect had led to their loss; there is, of course, no means of estimating their number. On this basis, 82 per cent of those examined in Salisbury and 66 per cent in Darlington showed evidence of past conservative treatment of

SALISBURY

Proportion decayed	Sex		Age-groups								Social class				All groups
	Males	Females	21-5	26-30	31-5	36-40	41-5	46-50	51-5	Over 55	I and II	III non-manual	III manual	IV and V	
Number	91	92	34	23	31	29	21	18	13	14	40	47	76	20	183
	Percentages														
None	26	30	21	—	23	14	29	39	23	57	40	32	22	15	28
Up to one-third	62	65	65	39	68	76	71	61	62	29	53	64	66	75	63
Over one-third and up to two-thirds	11	4	15	57	10	7	—	—	15	7	8	4	9	10	8
Over two-thirds	1	1	—	4	1	3	—	—	—	7	—	—	3	—	1
	100	100	100	100	100	100	100	100	100	100	100	100	100	100	100

DARLINGTON

Proportion decayed	Sex		Age-groups								Social class				All groups
	Males	Females	21-5	26-30	31-5	36-40	41-5	46-50	51-5	Over 55	I and II	III non-manual	III manual	IV and V	
Number	102	97	34	36	30	27	23	17	11	21	27	40	91	40	199[1]
	Percentages														
None	18	26	—	33	27	30	9	6	18	14	37	38	14	13	22
Up to one-third	73	65	21	61	60	59	83	88	73	71	52	55	78	73	69
Over one-third and up to two-thirds	9	8	71	6	13	11	6	9	9	9	7	8	7	15	8
Over two-thirds	1	1	9	—	—	—	4	—	—	5	4	—	1	—	1
	100	100	100	100	100	100	100	100	100	100	100	100	100	100	100

1. Because of imprecise occupational data one person could not be classified by social class.
N.B. This table relates only to those who still have some of their own teeth standing.

TABLE 11.4. *Proportion of teeth present found to be decayed*

	Males		Females		All persons	
Number	160[1]	202[1]	155	207	315	409
Percentages						
Subject has:						
No teeth present	43	50	41	53	42	51
No restorations	13	18	8	15	10	17
Up to one-third of teeth restored	24	22	23	14	23	18
Over one-third and up to two-thirds restored	19	10	26	16	22	13
Over two-thirds of teeth restored	3	—	3	1	3	—
	100	100	100	100	100	100

1. Roman figures represent Salisbury and italic figures Darlington.

TABLE II.5. *Restored teeth*

their teeth. In terms of the estimated total population this works out at about 13,500 persons in Salisbury and 17,500 in Darlington, not including children and teenagers. It is interesting that the difference between these two figures, 4,000, is only half the difference between the untreated decay figures for the two towns. Although decay figures are independent of the number of dentists available, restoration figures must depend directly on the number of dentists giving general dental treatment. This discrepancy therefore suggests a connection with the differing dentist/population ratios in the two areas.

In both towns about 40 per cent of all subjects had restorations in up to one-third of their teeth, but in Salisbury 42 per cent had more than one-third restored, compared with only 28 per cent in Darlington. The highest proportions with no restorations present were, as expected, found in the older age-groups who had lost most of their posterior teeth. These teeth are the ones most commonly attacked by decay and therefore the most likely to be filled.

Women tended to have more restored teeth than men in both towns, fewer women than men had received no restorative treatment at all and more women than men had over one-third of their teeth restored.

Social status was again a discriminating factor. In Salisbury 10

Proportion restored	Sex		Age-group								Social class				All groups
	Males	Females	21-5	26-30	31-5	36-40	41-5	46-50	51-5	Over 55	I and II	III non-manual	III manual	IV and V	
SALISBURY															
Number	92	91	34	23	31	29	21	18	13	14	40	47	76	20	183
	Percentages														
None	22	13	15	4	23	17	5	22	15	50	10	9	25	25	17
Up to one-third	41	38	41	39	42	45	29	56	38	21	18	49	41	60	40
Over one-third and up to two-thirds	33	44	41	57	35	31	67	17	31	14	58	43	33	10	38
Over two-thirds	4	4	3	—	—	7	—	6	15	14	15	—	1	5	5
	100	100	100	100	100	100	100	100	100	100	100	100	100	100	100
DARLINGTON															
Number	102	97	34	36	30	27	23	17	11	21	27	40	91	40	199[1]
	Percentages														
None	36	33	29	25	33	11	35	53	55	67	11	5	44	60	35
Up to one-third	44	31	29	42	33	52	48	35	45	19	33	48	38	28	38
Over one-third and up to two-thirds	20	34	41	33	33	33	17	6	—	14	48	48	18	13	27
Over two-thirds	—	2	—	—	—	4	—	6	—	—	7	—	—	—	1
	100	100	100	100	100	100	100	100	100	100	100	100	100	100	100

1. Because of imprecise occupational data one person could not be classified by social class.
N.B. This table relates only to those who still have some of their own teeth standing.

TABLE 11.6. *Proportion of teeth found to have been restored*

per cent in Classes I and II had no restored teeth and 73 per cent had over one-third restored while the figures for Classes IV and V were 25 and 15 per cent. In Darlington 11 per cent of Classes I and II had no restored teeth and 55 per cent had over one-third restored, while Classes IV and V contained 60 per cent with no restorations and only 13 per cent with over one-third restored.

Restorations in materials other than amalgam or silicate were rare. Only 10 gold inlays and 2 gold crowns were seen in Salisbury and 6 gold inlays and no gold crowns in Darlington. Two anterior jacket crowns were seen in Salisbury and 3 in Darlington. It is interesting that apart from 3 'private' gold inlays in Salisbury the inlays and crowns were all seen in the mouths of N.H.S. patients, and were evenly distributed throughout the social strata.

Before leaving dental conditions to consider periodontal disease it is perhaps useful to present an assessment of over-all dental health based on the number of sound teeth present, whether restored or not. In this analysis, 'good' means virtually no teeth missing and no teeth in need of restoration or extractions; 'fair' means either enough teeth missing to render a prosthesis desirable or more than one tooth actively decayed, or both; and 'poor' means more than half the normal number of teeth missing, or more than two-thirds of the standing teeth decayed, or both. On this basis only 5 per cent of the total sample examined in each area could be rated as being in good dental health. Thirty per cent in Salisbury, 25 per cent in Darlington were 'fair' and 64 per cent in Salisbury, 69 per cent in Darlington 'poor'. By definition, of course, all full denture wearers must be classified as 'poor'. Therefore, in both areas only 1 adult in every 20 could be said to have a fully functional, sound, natural dentition. In both towns about 20 per cent of the under-30s were rated as 'good' but the percentage fell rapidly to nil by the age of 45 in Salisbury and 40 in Darlington. The 'poor' percentage showed a marked rise after the age of 45 in Salisbury, 40 in Darlington, being 76–7 per cent at these ages and over 90 per cent by the age of 55 in Salisbury, 50 in Darlington. There was very little difference between men and women but social status differences were significant. In Salisbury 11 per cent of Classes I and II were 'good' and 46 per

cent 'poor' while 2 per cent of Classes IV and V were 'good' and
76 per cent 'poor'. In Darlington the figures were 18 and 55 per
cent for Classes I and II, and 1 and 84 per cent for Classes IV and V.

Periodontal disease

Periodontal disease attacks first the gums and then the bone which
supports the teeth. Its onset is insidious, the only symptoms
frequently being bleeding from the gums when brushed and a
'puffiness' of the gums around the teeth. There is usually no pain.
If, however, this condition is allowed to continue untreated the
whole of the supporting structure of the tooth will be destroyed
and the tooth lost as inevitably as if it had been riddled with decay.
More teeth are probably lost through gum disease than through
dental decay, which has usually done its worst by the time the
age of 35 has been reached. Periodontal disease, however, will
continue for as long as the tooth is present.

One of the initial causes of periodontal disease is the accumula-
tion of debris and the deposition of calculus or 'tartar' around the
necks of the teeth. This irritates the gums which become inflamed
and infected, and a process of recession occurs in which a deep
pocket develops between the gum and the tooth, full of infected
material which cannot now be removed by ordinary tooth
brushing and spreads slowly down the root of the tooth. The
presence and degree of disease present may therefore be assessed
by considering: (*a*) the amount of calculus present around the
teeth, (*b*) the degree of inflammation of the gums, and (*c*) the
degree of pocketing around the teeth. In the normal healthy
periodontium a shallow pocket exists, so in the periodontal
examination pockets were not considered to be pathological
unless they exceeded a depth of 3 mm. Inflammation, calculus,
and pocketing were assessed on a regional basis, each standing
tooth being checked for all three.

In order to simplify reporting, the periodontal state is recorded
in one of three grades; 'good', 'fair', and 'poor'. 'Good' means
that either little or no calculus and inflammation are present and
there are no inflammatory pockets around the teeth. 'Fair' means

that calculus and inflammation are more widespread and pocketing if present exists on no more than one tooth. 'Poor' implies
general inflammation and pathological pocketing on more than
two teeth. In terms of treatment, a 'good' case will require at the
most a routine scale and polish, a 'fair' case will require more
prolonged but still routine treatment, and a 'poor' case will either
need surgical treatment or else be beyond the stage where remedial
treatment is possible. To qualify for a 'good' rating, at least two-
thirds of the normal dentition must be standing. If less than one-
third are standing, the grading must inevitably be 'poor' since it
must be assumed that some teeth have been lost through periodontal disease.

In Salisbury only 18 per cent and in Darlington only 15 per
cent of the total sample examined—full denture wearers included
—could be graded as in 'good' periodontal health. A further 15
per cent in each town were 'fair' and the remainder, about 70 per
cent, 'poor'. In Salisbury 50 per cent were 'good' up to the age of
30, but the proportion fell rapidly to nil at the age of 55. In
Darlington the total started falling rapidly after the age of 25 and
was down to nil soon after the age of 50. From these ages onwards
the totals were virtually 100 per cent 'poor' in both towns.

Women were in a slightly better state than men by an equal
margin in each town. In Salisbury, for example, 14 per cent of the
men and 21 per cent of the women were 'good', and 69 per cent
of the men and 67 per cent of the women were 'bad'.

Social status differences were more marked in Salisbury than in
Darlington. In Darlington all the non-manual classes were graded
30 per cent 'good', 54 per cent 'bad', while the manual classes
were graded about 8 per cent 'good', 80 per cent 'bad'. In Salisbury
Classes I and II were graded in a manner similar to the Darlington
non-manual classes, but Classes IV and V were only 4 per cent
'good' and 83 per cent 'bad'.

Percentages excluding full denture wearers are given on p. 34.

Expressing these figures again in terms of the total population,
Salisbury had an estimated 10,300 adults with teeth of their own
in need of advanced periodontal treatment and a further 5,500 in
need of routine treatment while in Darlington 16,000 adults were

estimated to need advanced treatment and a further 12,500 to need routine treatment.

Dentures

In this section, 'full dentures' means full upper and lower dentures replacing all the natural teeth. A 'full' upper denture with a 'partial' lower denture is classified as a 'partial denture', since some natural teeth remain.

Out of every 10 adults examined in Salisbury, 4 wore full dentures, 2 wore partial dentures, and the remainder wore neither. Out of every 10 adults seen in Darlington, 5 wore full dentures, just over 1 wore partials, and just under 4 wore neither. In Darlington 4 per cent more women than men wore full dentures and 4 per cent less wore none, but in Salisbury there was no apparent difference between men and women.

In Salisbury, full dentures were found most frequently from the age of 45 onwards, becoming especially common (80 per cent) after the age of 55. In Darlington they were found most frequently after the age of 40, and reached 80 per cent of the total by the age of 50. The proportion of partial dentures worn was at its maximum (23–35 per cent) in Salisbury between the ages of 25 and 55, and in Darlington (14–22 per cent) between the ages of 25 and 45.

	Males		Females		All persons	
Number	97[1]	*123*[1]	97	*133*	194	*256*
Percentages						
Full upper and lower	69	*79*	66	*80*	68	*80*
Full upper only	2	*6*	3	*7*	3	*6*
Full upper and partial lower	6	*4*	6	*3*	6	*4*
Partial upper and lower	7	*3*	12	*2*	10	*3*
Partial upper	13	*7*	9	*7*	11	*7*
Partial lower	1	*1*	1	—	1	—
'Spoon' denture	1	*1*	2	*1*	2	*1*
	100	*100*	100	*100*	100	*100*

1. Roman figures represent Salisbury and italic figures Darlington.

TABLE 11.7. *Type of denture possessed. Denture-wearers*

	Males		Females		All persons	
Number	160[1]	202[1]	155	207	315	409
Percentages						
Require dentures	21	21	14	18	17	20
Present dentures inadequate	4	3	6	3	5	3
Total needing new dentures	25	24	20	21	22	23

1. Roman figures represent Salisbury and italic figures Darlington.

TABLE II.8. *Denture requirements*

The most commonly worn partial denture patterns in Salisbury were partial upper only and partial upper/partial lower followed by full upper/partial lower. In Darlington the most common were partial upper only and full upper only followed by full upper/ partial lower and partial upper/partial lower.

In any population group there will always be a number of people who while needing dentures either cannot tolerate them or have never bothered to obtain them. There will also be others content to wear inadequate dentures; for example, a partial upper denture worn when all upper teeth have been lost. This problem is not just one of aesthetics, for unless some form of dentition exists food must either be bolted down or else mashed into a 'pap', and neither form of intake is either satisfying or in all probability ideal for the healthy human digestion. In Salisbury 17 per cent of the examined sample needed dentures, considerably more men than women and 5 per cent wore inadequate dentures, slightly more women than men. In Darlington 20 per cent needed dentures, slightly more men than women, and 3 per cent wore inadequate dentures. In terms of the total population, 6,100 in Salisbury and 12,400 in Darlington were estimated to need new dentures for these reasons.

Many people wear dentures quite contentedly which a dentist would consider to be misfits. The most common cause of badly fitting dentures is probably failure of the wearer to have them replaced when they no longer conform to the mouth contours. No denture can be expected to last indefinitely, but many people

TABLE II.9. *Prosthetic conditions*

Subject has:	Sex		Age-groups											Social class				
	Males	Females	21–5	26–30	31–5	36–40	41–5	46–50	51–5	56–60	61–5	66–70	Over 70	I and II	III non-manual	III manual	IV and V	All groups
SALISBURY																		
Number	160	155	37	23	35	38	31	35	23	25	30	12	26	56	71	142	46	315
	Percentages																	
No dentures	39	37	86	65	66	45	42	23	30	12	7	—	4	55	45	30	35	28
Partial dentures	19	21	5	35	23	32	26	29	26	8	10	17	8	16	21	24	11	20
Full dentures	42	41	8	—	11	24	32	49	43	80	83	83	88	29	34	46	54	42
	100	100	100	100	100	100	100	100	100	100	100	100	100	100	100	100	100	100
DARLINGTON																		
Number	202	207	34	39	35	36	49	47	50	36	28	22	33	40	71	193	104	409[1]
	Percentages																	
No dentures	39	36	91	74	57	61	29	34	12	8	14	27	6	48	39	38	31	37
Partial dentures	13	13	9	21	29	14	22	2	10	9	11	5	6	20	20	9	12	13
Full dentures	48	52	—	5	14	25	49	64	78	83	75	68	88	32	41	53	58	50
	100	100	100	100	100	100	100	100	100	100	100	100	100	100	100	100	100	100

1. Because of imprecise occupational data one person could not be classified by social class.

C

	Partial		Full	
Number	63[1]	52[1]	131	*204*
Percentages				
Satisfactory	63	*75*	36	*58*
Unsatisfactory (upper or				
lower only)	14	*6*	34	*24*
Unsatisfactory	16	*17*	27	*16*
No information available	6	*2*	2	*2*
	100	*100*	100	*100*

1. Roman figures represent Salisbury and italic figures Darlington.

TABLE II.10. *Fit of denture. Denture wearers*

seem to think that they should! Another cause of badly fitting dentures is improper cleaning methods, including overheating. In assessing the fit of dentures in the course of this survey, the dental examiner's standards were not exacting. The fit of a denture was only graded as 'bad' if the upper denture fell down as soon as the mouth was opened or if with the denture firmly in position there was still more than a quarter of an inch of 'play' possible. It was found that only 36 per cent of the full dentures seen in Salisbury could be considered a good fit and only 58 per cent of those seen in Darlington. It should be remembered, however, that especially in lower dentures a good fit is sometimes impossible to obtain because of the lack of suitable gum ridges to support the denture. A further 34 per cent of the full denture wearers in Salisbury had well-fitting upper dentures but poorly fitting lowers, the figure for Darlington being 24 per cent. No information was available on 2 per cent of denture wearers in both towns whose dentures were not available for inspection at the time of the examination. 63 per cent in Salisbury, 75 per cent in Darlington of all partial dentures seen were a good fit, and in 14 per cent (Salisbury), 6 per cent (Darlington) one part was satisfactory while the other was not. No information was possible on 6 per cent in Salisbury, 2 per cent in Darlington of the partial denture wearers, since the dentures were not available for inspection.

In both towns 9 out of 10 full dentures seen were made entirely of acrylic plastic. One set in each town was made of acrylic and stainless steel and the remainder were made of vulcanite. 85–90 per cent of partial dentures were made of acrylic, 13 per cent in Salisbury, 10 per cent in Darlington were made of acrylic and gold or stainless steel, and 6 per cent in Darlington were made of vulcanite.

Dentures were checked to see whether they were cracked or had missing teeth or flanges. Three out of every 10 sets of full dentures seen in Salisbury were unsatisfactory in this respect and 2 out of every 10 in Darlington. Two out of every 10 in Salisbury, and 3 out of 10 in Darlington of the partials were similarly unsatisfactory. Proportionally more women than men had unsatisfactory dentures for these reasons, although more men than women had badly fitting dentures. Under 5 per cent of the total number of denture wearers seen said that they regularly used a proprietary denture fixative. Nine upper dentures in the Salisbury sample and 20 in Darlington were fitted with a button for the attachment of a rubber suction-pad, although in only 4 of these dentures in Salisbury, 3 in Darlington, was the actual suction pad in position. In these cases there were signs of palatal inflammation or damage, and in one case, in Darlington, where the pad had been in constant use for many years, it appeared that the palate was almost perforated.

Inquiries concerning denture-wearing habits suggested that in Salisbury 37 per cent of full denture wearers wore their dentures all night compared with 51 per cent in Darlington. Fifty-five per cent (Salisbury), 43 per cent (Darlington) wore their dentures during the day only. Fifty per cent (Salisbury), 60 per cent (Darlington) of the partial denture wearers claimed to wear their dentures continually, and 29 per cent (Salisbury), 25 per cent (Darlington) said they wore them only during the day. The remainder either wore their dentures irregularly or not at all. However, these figures need to be considered bearing in mind that many people who claimed to wear their dentures continually had such ill-fitting sets that it was difficult to see how they could possibly eat or even talk with them in, while others making a similar claim were not wearing their dentures when the examiner called.

About 90 per cent of all dentures seen appeared to be looked after well, although only 70 per cent of the Salisbury partials were. Cleaning methods were not investigated in detail but it became clear that the most popular cleaning agent, in Darlington especially, was a well-known brand of household bleach.

Questioning of owners gave the age of 40 per cent of all full dentures in both towns as being under 5 years and 30 per cent as being over 15 years. Fifty per cent of the partials were under 5 years old and 55 per cent (Salisbury), 10 per cent (Darlington) were over 15 years. Since these figures rely on a person's recollection of a relatively obscure event, they must not be considered as particularly accurate.

One interesting fact emerging from this denture examination was the number of people in both towns who were not wearing their latest dentures. The classic examples of this were the elderly people, who having worn a vulcanite denture for 15 or more years finally decided to have a new set made. However, they had become so used to the old ones that the new set seemed to be 'much too tight' and so were relegated to the dresser drawer while the old ones, considered dentally as loose, ill-fitting, and useless, were still preferred.

To summarize the denture state of the sample populations examined, in Salisbury 38 per cent either did not need dentures or were satisfactorily fitted out with them, and 62 per cent or approximately 17,300, needed dentures or were wearing unsatisfactory sets. In Darlington 47 per cent did not need dentures or else wore satisfactory sets, and 53 per cent, or approximately 28,500 needed them.

Summary of dental data

To conclude this section, data on dental, periodontal, and prosthetic conditions have been combined by the method indicated in the Appendix D on oral health grading to provide information on general oral health. As a result, only 4 per cent in both towns could be said to be in a healthy, natural, oral state. The remaining 96 per cent either needed dental treatment or had passed the stage where treatment other than the provision of full dentures could benefit them. No one over the age of 35 could be said to be in a state of absolute oral health.

In the next section of this report, these data will be compared with people's own assessments of their dental conditions, as a preliminary to investigating general attitudes towards dentistry and dental treatment.

III

Sociological data

1. Dental comparisons

It was clearly important to discover what the average person thought of his or her own oral state, since this bears directly on the demand for dental treatment. One man may consider that his teeth are in a healthy condition if he is not actually suffering from toothache while another may be worried by staining on his otherwise perfect teeth. This 'dental comparison' section explores these self-assessments and compares them with the oral states reported by the dental examiner. Only data on those both interviewed and examined are included, and data on standing teeth will not include full denture wearers.

Condition of teeth present

Everyone except full denture wearers was asked 'What state do you think your own teeth are in now?' and the possible answers were classified as 'very good', 'good', 'fair', 'poor', and 'don't know'. There were only two 'don't knows' in Salisbury and none in Darlington, so that almost everyone asked, clearly felt themselves competent to answer the question. Table III.1 shows the relationship between these personal assessments and those made by the dental examiner, using the dental summary given on p. 20. Actual numbers are given, as the 'fair' and 'poor' groups are so small as to make percentages misleading. One glance at this table shows that the majority took a far more optimistic view of their dental health than did the examiner. In both towns 60–70 per cent

Objective assessment	Subjective assessment Very good and good	Fair	Poor	Don't know	All subjects
Good	14[1] 20[1]	2 2	1 —	1 —	18 22
Fair	60 80	30 20	7 4	— —	97 104
Poor	40 34	19 27	9 11	1 —	69 72
All subjects	114 134	51 49	17 15	2 —	184 198

(Table does not include full denture wearers.)

1. Roman figures represent Salisbury and italic figures Darlington.

TABLE III.1. *Subjective and objective assessments of dental health compared*

of the total thought their teeth were in 'very good' or 'good' condition, 25–30 per cent thought they were in 'fair' condition, and only 5–10 per cent thought they were in 'poor' condition, yet the examiner considered that only 10–11 per cent were in 'good' condition, 52–53 per cent were in 'fair' condition, and 36–37 per cent in 'poor' condition. He agreed with only 10–15 per cent of those who considered that their teeth were 'very good' or 'good' and considered the teeth of a further 25–35 per cent to be 'poor'. He agreed with 60 per cent in Salisbury, 40 per cent in Darlington of the self-assessed 'fairs', and thought that about 5 per cent of this group had been too severe on themselves, although it must be remembered that 5 per cent was actually only two individuals in each area! He agreed with all the self-assessed 'poors' except for 8 individuals in Salisbury (47 per cent) and 4 in Darlington (27 per cent). Therefore, by the examiner's criteria, 30 per cent (Salisbury), 25 per cent (Darlington) assessed their dental health correctly, 5 per cent were too pessimistic and 65 per cent (Salisbury), 70 per cent (Darlington) too optimistic.

Unfortunately we can only guess at the criteria people used in arriving at these self-assessments. Clearly they bore no relation to those used by the examiner since the proportions of 'good', 'fair', and 'poor' examiner assessments are nearly constant for each of the three self-assessment totals. A similar relationship exists when tooth loss, decay, or conservative treatment data are compared

	Very good		Good		Fair		Poor	
Number	46[1]	60[1]	68	74	51	49	17	15
Percentages								
Number of teeth found present								
20–32	76	87	62	70	63	53	47	47
12–19	11	12	28	15	31	24	41	20
0–11	13	2	10	15	6	22	12	33
	100	100	100	100	100	100	100	100
Proportion of teeth decayed								
None	39	27	31	24	18	18	12	33
Up to one-third	57	70	59	70	76	67	59	53
Over one-third and up to two-thirds	4	3	9	4	6	14	18	13
Over two-thirds	—	—	—	1	—	—	12	—
	100	100	100	100	100	100	100	100
Proportion of teeth restored								
None	28	18	18	35	6	41	23	73
Up to one-third	41	47	36	32	41	41	47	20
Over one-third and up to two-thirds	30	32	42	32	49	18	12	7
Over two-thirds	—	3	4	—	4	—	18	—
	100	100	100	100	100	100	100	100

1. Roman figures represent Salisbury and italic Darlington.

TABLE III.2. *Self-assessed dental condition analysed by objective dental data*

individually with self-assessments, although there is some evidence that tooth loss was at least a significant factor to some people.

Periodontal condition

People with teeth of their own remaining were asked, 'How would you describe the state of your gums?', with possible answers of 'healthy', 'fair', 'poor', and 'don't know'. Everyone asked was prepared to answer this question—there were no 'don't knows' in either town. Table III.3 shows the relationship between these assessments and the dental examiner's findings given on p. 34 and again actual numbers are used for the same reasons as before. Optimism here was even greater than with the dental assessments. In both towns 90–5 per cent thought that their gums were

Objective assessment	Subjective assessment						
	Healthy		Fair		Poor		All subjects
Good	53[1]	59[1]	2	—	—	—	55 59
Fair	44	61	—	2	—	—	44 63
Poor	66	70	13	4	6	2	85 76
All subjects	163	190	15	6	6	2	184 198

(Table excludes those with full dentures.)

1. Roman figures represent Salisbury and italic figures Darlington.

TABLE III.3. *Subjective and objective assessments of periodontal health compared*

'healthy' and less than 5 per cent thought that their gums were in 'poor' condition. The examiner considered that 30 per cent in both towns had 'healthy' gums, 25–30 per cent had 'fair' gums, and 40–5 per cent 'poor' gums. He agreed with 31–2 per cent of those who considered that their gums were 'healthy' and judged the periodontal condition of a further 37–40 per cent to be 'poor'. He agreed with only two of the 'fairs' (in Darlington), but thought that two more (in Salisbury) had been too severe in their assessment. He agreed with the eight people in both areas who considered that their gums were in a bad state. Therefore using the examiner's criteria, 32 per cent in both towns judged their periodontal state correctly. Sixty-seven per cent were too optimistic and 0–1 per cent were too pessimistic.

It could be argued that since the examiner included the loss of teeth in arriving at his periodontal assessment, and since this factor was almost certainly not considered by members of the sample in answering the question, comparison of the two assessments is unfair. It was found, however, that in almost every case where enough teeth had been lost to affect the periodontal grading the state of the remaining periodontium justified the grade given. In other words healthy gums were very rare in a mouth from which many teeth had been lost.

These data seem to indicate that the average person has little if any idea of the meaning of periodontal disease, or the part it plays in oral health. The significance of these findings will be discussed in the final part of this Report.

Full dentures

Denture wearers were asked, 'Have you any complaints about your dentures?' and in both towns 80–5 per cent of full denture wearers said that they had no complaints. Of the remainder, 60–70 per cent said that their dentures did not fit and the rest gave aesthetic reasons for their dissatisfaction. Therefore 11 per cent of the full denture wearers interviewed and examined were dissatisfied with the fit of their dentures. In the opinion of the dental examiner, however, only 36 per cent of the full dentures seen in Salisbury and 60 per cent of those seen in Darlington were a good fit. An analysis of the two opinions is shown in the following table:

	Salisbury	Darlington
Considered a good fit by examiner and wearer	35% (46)	56% (114)
Considered a bad fit by examiner and wearer	11% (14)	7% (15)
Considered a good fit by wearer only	53% (70)	32% (65)
Considered a good fit by examiner only	1% (1)	4% (8)

Actual figures are given in parentheses.

Denture wearers were clearly far more tolerant about the fit of their dentures than was the examiner. One reason for this has already been mentioned; people become used to a set of dentures and prefer a familiar bad fit to an unfamiliar good fit. It was significant that in both towns the majority of dissatisfied denture wearers had done nothing to have their complaints remedied. It is also difficult to judge the 'honesty' of the answers given to this question. Admitting to having badly fitting dentures, especially after some years of wear, is to some extent an admission of failure to cope with the problem of dentures, and reluctance on this score would be only natural, especially if the answer had to be given in

	Nos.		Percentage in groups A		B		C	
Last visit								
6 months or under	109[1]	*104*[1]	75	*89*	16	*8*	9	*3*
Over 6 months to 1 year	36	*28*	75	*79*	11	*14*	14	*7*
Over 1 year to 2 years	48	*53*	75	*91*	13	*6*	13	*3*
Over 2 years to 5 years	94	*116*	68	*78*	17	*16*	15	*6*
Over 5 years to 10 years	63	*79*	67	*67*	16	*19*	17	*14*
Over 10 years to 15 years	34	*43*	65	*81*	6	*—*	29	*19*
Over 15 years	78	*87*	53	*71*	14	*16*	33	*13*
D.K./no visit	3	*6*	≠	*≠*	≠	*≠*	≠	*≠*
Type of dental service used								
N.H.S.	348	*372*	75	*84*	13	*10*	12	*6*
Private	42	*62*	45	*66*	24	*18*	31	*16*
Not been since 1948	73	*78*	48	*69*	15	*17*	37	*14*
Both N.H.S. and private	2	*4*	≠	*≠*	≠	*≠*	≠	*≠*
Denture status								
No dentures	146	*183*	73	*81*	18	*10*	9	*9*
Partial dentures	118	*78*	66	*72*	15	*18*	19	*10*
Full dentures	201	*255*	65	*80*	11	*12*	24	*8*
Self-assessment of state teeth in now								
F.D./no teeth	206	*266*	64	*79*	13	*12*	24	*9*
Very good	61	*71*	75	*85*	7	*13*	18	*3*
Good	97	*92*	70	*80*	19	*11*	11	*9*
Fair	71	*66*	72	*74*	14	*12*	14	*14*
Poor	27	*21*	63	*71*	30	*14*	7	*14*
Don't know	3	*—*	≠	*—*	≠	*—*	≠	*—*
Self-assessment of amount of treatment needed								
Now under treatment	22	*8*	77	*≠*	14	*≠*	9	*≠*
None	276	*312*	64	*81*	13	*11*	22	*8*
Some	126	*165*	77	*79*	13	*12*	10	*10*
Lot	32	*22*	59	*55*	28	*32*	13	*14*
Don't know	9	*9*	≠	*≠*	≠	*≠*	≠	*≠*

Key: Group A = Originally agreed to dental examination and were examined.
Group B = Originally agreed to dental examination but were not examined.
Group C = Refused dental examination when interviewed.
≠ Indicates percentage too small to be significant.

1. Roman figures represent Salisbury and italic figures Darlington.

TABLE III.4. *Sociological data analysed by dental examination record*

the presence of other members of the family. But whatever factors affected the data obtained, it is clear that imperfectly fitting dentures were tolerated by a substantial proportion of denture wearers in both towns. It should again be stressed that in many of these cases, no improvement to the dentures was possible owing to the unfavourable anatomy of the wearer's mouth, and in fact poor design or workmanship were negligible factors. People clearly failed to realize that any denture has a limited life, the length of which depends on the state of the oral tissue when it was fitted. For example, a denture fitted immediately after all teeth have been lost may only last for a year, while a denture fitted 5 years later may with modification last for 15 or more years if it is checked every 5 years.

The significance of these subjective and objective comparisons will be discussed in the final part of the Report.

2. Dental attitudes and opinions

Visiting the dentist

Everyone interviewed in the survey was asked, 'When was your last visit to the dentist?', and the answers were grouped into categories ranging from 'less than 6 months ago' to 'over 15 years ago'. Grouping the samples in terms of age, social status, and denture status then produced some significant differences. Forty per cent (Salisbury), 30 per cent (Darlington) of the non-denture wearers said that they had visited a dentist within the past 6 months, and 85 per cent (Salisbury), 78 per cent (Darlington) claimed that they had been within the past 5 years. Only 1 per cent (Salisbury), 3 per cent (Darlington) of the total sample had never visited a dentist. On the other hand, only 5 per cent (Salisbury), 10 per cent (Darlington) of the full denture wearers had been within the past 6 months and only 36 per cent (Salisbury), 39 per cent (Darlington) within the past 5 years. These figures seem to confirm the suggestion made in the previous section that full denture wearers rarely return to a dentist after their dentures have been fitted. The visiting pattern of partial denture wearers was inconclusive, the majority having visited a dentist some time within the past 10 years.

The most recent dental attenders appeared to be the 26–30-year-olds. Seventy-five per cent (Salisbury), 57 per cent (Darlington) of this group claimed to have visited a dentist within the past year, and 86 per cent (Salisbury), 71 per cent (Darlington) within the past 2 years, compared with 73 per cent (Salisbury), 69 per cent (Darlington) of the 21–5-year-olds and 63 per cent (Salisbury), 47 per cent (Darlington) of the 31–5-year-olds. Most of those aged over 60 had not been to a dentist for more than 10 years. These figures give no reason for the last visit; that is whether it was an 'emergency' to have a tooth out or part of a routine course of conservative treatment, but they do indicate a peak demand for dental treatment below the age of 30 falling off slowly up to the age of 45 and rapidly thereafter.

The demand for dental treatment was also related to social status. Sixty-two per cent in Salisbury and 65 per cent in Darlington of Classes I and II said that they had been to a dentist within the past two years, but only 23 per cent (Salisbury), 31 per cent (Darlington) of Class V made the same claim. One difference between the two areas was that in Darlington there were no attendance variations within the 'manual' groupings while in Salisbury Class III manual showed more recent attendances than Class IV, and Class IV than Class V. In both towns all those claiming never to have visited a dentist were in Class V. In considering social status data, however, there may well be a slight bias since those in the 'higher' social classes possibly gave less reliable answers than those in the 'lower' classes. An individual in Classes I or II knows that he or she should visit a dentist every six months and may therefore be reluctant to admit to not having been for some time. A Class V individual, on the other hand, will probably feel less inhibited.

Subjects were also asked how often they had been to the dentist in the previous five years; whether 'regularly' (once a year or more), 'occasionally', 'rarely and only when in pain', 'rarely and only for new dentures or denture repairs', or 'never'. Taking the samples as a whole, 2 people out of every 5 had not visited a dentist at all, and only 1 out of 5 in Salisbury, 1 out of 10 in Darlington claimed to have attended regularly. About the same number went 'occasionally', 16 per cent in Salisbury and 25 per cent in Darlington went because they were in pain and 10 per cent (Salisbury), 13 per cent (Darlington) went with denture troubles. In terms of the total population, therefore, these data indicate that about 5,300 in Salisbury and 5,400 in Darlington visited a dentist 'regularly' during the five years previous to the survey. A further 4,500 in Salisbury and 13,500 in Darlington were 'emergency' patients and in pain. These figures probably reflect the difference in the number of dentists available as well as any 'attitude' differences between the two areas, and it is significant that with equal numbers of dentists available, the number of people claiming to attend regularly is also very similar in the two towns in spite of the population difference. It must be remembered that these figures do not include anyone under the age of 21. Significantly more women than men attend regularly, and fewer women attended as emergency patients. Was this because women cared for their teeth more than men, or was it because men had difficulty in obtaining time off from work to visit a dentist? Experience suggests the latter reason.

In terms of age, the 26–30 age-group attended most regularly for dental treatment, more so in Salisbury than in Darlington. Regular attendance in Salisbury averaged between 30 and 55 per cent in age-groups up to the age of 45 and then fell sharply. In Darlington regular attendance ranged between 20 and 35 per cent in age-groups up to the age of 40 and then fell off. From then on 'no visits' was the rule in nearly all age-groups. The 'emergency-pain' category produced percentages varying between 15 and 30 per cent in Salisbury for age-groups up to the age of 65, and between 40 and 50 per cent in Darlington for age-groups up to the age of 40, then falling off rapidly.

Social Classes I and II produced more professed regular attenders than the other classes, and more non-manual workers than manual workers claimed they attended regularly. Again it is difficult to say to what degree this is due to different social attitudes, how much to ease of obtaining leave of absence from work, and how much to misleading information. However, there is clearly a different approach to dental visits in manual and non-manual classes. Thirty-three per cent in Salisbury and 35 per cent in Darlington of Classes I and II claimed to have attended regularly compared with no-one in either town in Class V.

Only 21 per cent in Salisbury and 25 per cent in Darlington of the full-denture wearers had seen a dentist in connection with their dentures during the previous 5 years and 64 per cent (Salisbury), 61 per cent (Darlington) had not been to a dentist at all. This leaves a further 14 per cent in both towns who were presumably fitted with full dentures for the first time in this period, and of these 57 per cent (Salisbury), 71 per cent (Darlington) originally went because they were in pain.

Those who had been to a dentist within the past 5 years were asked why they went, and the answers given emphasize the area differences. In Salisbury the most common reason suggested (34 per cent) was for a routine check-up, but in Darlington the most frequently cited reason (40 per cent) was to have a tooth out. The second most frequently mentioned reason in both towns (28 per cent Salisbury, 35 per cent Darlington) was to have dentures

Total number of respondents answering questions	287[1]	301[1]
	Percentage giving reason	
Reason given		
Toothache or pain	19	29
Check up	34	23
Extraction(s)	24	40
Dentures—fitting of or repairs	28	35
Fillings	19	12
Other	8	2

(N.B. These percentages total more than 100 since some subjects listed more than one reason.)

1. Roman figures represent Salisbury and italic figures Darlington.

TABLE III.7. *Reasons given for last visit to the dentist*

fitted or repaired, and the third, 'having a tooth out' in Salisbury (24 per cent), and 'toothache' in Darlington (29 per cent). There is some slight overlap in these figures since some people gave more than one reason for their last visit. In Darlington only 23 per cent of the sample mentioned a routine check-up as the reason for their last visit.

All those who claimed that they had visited a dentist at some time in their lives and who still had some teeth left were asked when they next expected to have to visit the dentist. Forty-five per cent (Salisbury), 37 per cent (Darlington) replied 'within 6 months'. These percentages were higher for men than women, and higher for younger people than for older. They reflected fairly accurately the past 'regular' attenders, and included 86 per cent (Salisbury), 93 per cent (Darlington) of those who said they had been regular attenders in the past. Only 8 per cent (Salisbury), 12 per cent (Darlington) of those who had not visited a dentist for 5 years but still had some teeth said that they would probably have to visit one within 6 months. This seems to bear out the optimistic subjective view of oral health reported in the previous section.

The National Health Service and private treatment

Only 9 per cent in Salisbury and 12 per cent in Darlington of the adult population interviewed said that they usually went to a private dentist, and a further 16 per cent (Salisbury), 15 per cent (Darlington) had not been to a dentist since the introduction of the N.H.S. The remainder said that they usually received their dental treatment under N.H.S. conditions. More men than women received private treatment in both areas, but age differences provided few points of contrast other than a tendency for the proportion seeking private treatment to be lowest in the under-30 age-group in both areas.

Social class variations were slight, but the proportions seeking private treatment were perhaps surprisingly highest in Class V in Salisbury, Classes IV and V in Darlington, and lowest in all the non-manual classes in both Salisbury and Darlington. It is of

D

	No dentures		Partial dentures		Full dentures		All groups	
Number	138[1]	165[1]	112	70	142	203	392	438
Percentages								
Types of service usually used								
N.H.S.	88	75	88	89	90	92	89	85
Both N.H.S. and private	1	1	—	1	1	—	1	1
Private	12	24	12	10	9	8	11	14
	100	100	100	100	100	100	100	100

(N.B. Those who have not been to the dentist since the introduction of N.H.S. have been excluded from this table.)

1. Roman figures represent Salisbury and italic figures Darlington.

TABLE III.10. *Type of dental service used analysed by denture status*

interest that 79 per cent of all the private patients interviewed came from the manual classes and only 29 per cent from the non-manual classes in both areas.

Seventy-nine per cent (Salisbury), 76 per cent (Darlington) of all private patients had had some experience of N.H.S. dentistry. When asked why they preferred to be treated privately, the usual reason, given by about three-quarters of the professed 'private' attenders, was that they received better service privately with less waiting both for an appointment and in the waiting-room, and also more personal attention. Less waiting-time was a point made especially by manual workers who presumably lost more money the longer they were away from work. The next most common reason for having private treatment (14 per cent Salisbury, 26 per cent Darlington), and this was most common among full denture wearers, was that treatment, as opposed to service, was better. Finally, 10 per cent in Salisbury, 3 per cent in Darlington said that they received private treatment because they had stayed with their own dentist when the N.H.S. was introduced, and he had not joined the scheme. Private patients, however, were no more liable to be regular attenders than N.H.S. patients.

On the question of changing dentists, 74 per cent in Salisbury, and 69 per cent in Darlington, of those who had visited a dentist within the past 5 years said that they had a 'regular' dentist.

Ninety-two per cent in Salisbury, 94 per cent in Darlington went to a dentist practising within the survey area.

One surprising finding was that only 5 per cent of those interviewed in both areas had ever been treated by a female dentist. Many people expressed surprise at the existence of women in the profession, but 42 per cent in Salisbury and 51 per cent in Darlington said that they would not mind if their dentist were a man or a woman.

Dentures

Some purely dental data on denture-wearing and denture-fitting have been presented in previous sections, and it is the purpose now to deal with the social aspects of denture-wearing. Remembering that more people were interviewed than were examined, it should be noted that of the total adult sample interviewed, 43 per cent in Salisbury and 49 per cent in Darlington wore full upper and lower dentures, and 25 per cent in Salisbury and 15 per cent in Darlington wore partial dentures. In terms of the total adult population this averages roughly 12,000 full denture wearers and 7,000 partial denture wearers in Salisbury, and 26,000 full denture wearers and 8,000 partial denture wearers in Darlington. Five people in Salisbury and 11 in Darlington had lost all their teeth but did not have any dentures.

In both towns, considerably more full denture wearers than non-wearers complained of having had 'some' or a 'lot' of trouble from their teeth and gums, and conversely fewer said that they had experienced 'little' trouble. Of course it must be remembered that full denture wearers were generally older than non-wearers and had therefore had a longer time in which to suffer.

Full denture wearers in both towns generally denied that they had any trouble eating with their dentures. Answers to the question, 'How often do teeth or dentures cause you trouble when eating?' were graded 'never', 'sometimes', and 'often', and in Salisbury, for example, 80 per cent of the full denture wearers said that they 'never' had trouble eating and only 4 per cent said that they 'often' had trouble. In the same town 83 per cent of

	Males		Females		Total sample	
Number	208[1]	236[1]	257	280	465	516
Percentages						
Subject has trouble when eating						
Never	80	82	81	81	80	80
Sometimes	17	16	16	16	16	16
Often	3	2	4	4	3	4
	100	100	100	100	100	100

1. Roman figures represent Salisbury and italic figures Darlington.

TABLE III.11. *Dental troubles when eating*

	No dentures		Partial dentures		Full dentures		All groups	
Number	146[1]	183[1]	118	78	201	255	465	516
Percentages								
Trouble in eating								
Never	83	90	78	87	80	73	80	80
Sometimes	16	10	18	12	16	22	16	16
Often	1	1	4	1	4	5	3	4
	100	100	100	100	100	100	100	100

1. Roman figures represent Salisbury and italic figures Darlington.

TABLE III.12. *Self-assessment of trouble in eating analysed by denture status*

those with no dentures said that they 'never' had trouble eating and 1 per cent said they 'often' had trouble. The figures are nearly the same in Darlington, 73 per cent of the full denture wearers 'never' had any trouble and 5 per cent 'often' had trouble compared with 90 and 1 per cent respectively of the non-denture wearers. Clearly 'trouble eating' means different things to different people.

About 40 per cent of all persons interviewed in both areas had been wearing dentures for more than 15 years, 16 per cent for 5–15 years and 10 per cent for less than 5 years.

Those without dentures were asked if the thought of wearing dentures ever bothered them, and in both areas 45 per cent of those asked said 'yes'. A further 51 per cent in Salisbury, and 45

	Bothers		Doesn't bother		Don't know		All groups	
Number	66[1]	*83*[1]	74	*82*	6	*18*	146	*183*
Expectations of denture needs	Percentages							
Expects to need them	55	*19*	55	*44*	≠	*22*	55	*31*
Hopes not to need them	29	*63*	18	*43*	≠	*61*	23	*54*
Doesn't expect to need them	12	*11*	20	*10*	≠	*11*	16	*10*
Don't know	5	*7*	7	*4*	≠	*6*	7	*5*
	100	*100*	100	*100*	≠	*100*	100	*100*

≠ Indicates numbers too small for percentage to be significant.

1. Roman figures represent Salisbury and italic figures Darlington.

TABLE III.15. *Thoughts about wearing dentures analysed by expectations of denture needs*

per cent in Darlington said that the thought of wearing dentures did not worry them, and 4 per cent in Salisbury, and 10 per cent in Darlington did not know what to think. Considerably more women than men viewed the onset of full dentures with misgiving, 57 per cent in Salisbury, 54 per cent in Darlington compared with only 34 per cent in Salisbury, 37 per cent in Darlington of the men. Age had little effect on this aspect of denture-wearing, although non-manual classes disliked the idea of wearing dentures more than manual classes. Those not wearing dentures were also asked, 'Do you think you will ever need dentures?' with answers graded as 'yes', 'hope not', 'no', and 'don't know'. Most people in Salisbury (55 per cent) expected to have to wear dentures while most people in Darlington (54 per cent) hoped they would not have to wear them. This is surprising in view of the higher prevalence of dentures in Darlington. Sixteen per cent in Salisbury did not expect to have to wear dentures, and 10 per cent in Darlington. Seven per cent in Salisbury, 5 per cent in Darlington were 'don't know'.

Assessments of oral health

Self-assessments of oral health have already been compared with the findings of the dental examiner, and in this section these self-assessments are considered in greater detail.

	No dentures		Partial dentures		Full dentures		All groups	
Number	146[1]	183[1]	118	78	201	255	465	516
Amount of trouble	Percentages							
Considerable	10	3	10	6	17	13	13	8
Some	14	7	28	12	31	25	25	17
Little	47	64	50	69	31	51	41	58
None	28	26	12	13	20	11	21	16
	100	100	100	100	100	100	100	100

1. Roman figures represent Salisbury and italic figures Darlington.

TABLE III.16. *Self-assessment of trouble from teeth and gums analysed by denture status*

Subjects were asked how much trouble their teeth and gums had been to them, with answers graded into 'none', 'a little', 'some', and 'a lot', and in both areas most people, 62 per cent in Salisbury and 74 per cent in Darlington, said that their teeth and gums had been 'little or no trouble'. Only 13 per cent in Salisbury, 8 per cent in Darlington complained of considerable trouble from their teeth and gums. However, when the groups were sub-divided according to denture status, an interesting pattern emerged. The percentages claiming little or no trouble were: non-denture wearers, 75 per cent in Salisbury and 90 per cent in Darlington; partial denture wearers, 62 per cent in Salisbury and 82 per cent in Darlington; the full denture wearers, 51 per cent in Salisbury and 62 per cent in Darlington. The suggestion seems to be that 'trouble' with teeth and gums is directly related by most people to tooth loss.

When asked how much dental treatment they thought they needed, most people (59 per cent in Salisbury, 60 per cent in Darlington), answered 'none'. Only 7 per cent in Salisbury, 4 per cent in Darlington thought they needed a 'lot' of treatment, and 2 per cent in both areas refused to hazard a guess. The 'no treatment required' verdict was most common in Salisbury among the over-40s and in Darlington among the over-30s. Of those not wearing full dentures, 40 per cent in both areas thought they needed 'no' treatment and 9 per cent in Salisbury, 7 per cent in

	None		Some		Considerable		Don't know		All groups	
Number	104[1]	105[1]	125	120	22	17	8	8	259	250
Self-assessed dental condition	Percentages									
Very good	34	40	20	22	5	6	≠	≠	24	28
Good	44	48	36	33	9	6	≠	≠	37	37
Fair	19	11	34	37	27	41	≠	≠	27	26
Poor	2	1	10	9	59	47	≠	≠	10	8
Don't know	1	—	—	—	—	—	≠	≠	1	—
	100	100	100	100	100	100	≠	≠	100	100

≠ Indicates numbers too small for percentage to be significant.

1. Roman figures represent Salisbury and italic figures Darlington.

TABLE III.17. *Amount of dental treatment thought to be needed analysed by self-assessment of dental conditions*

	Very good		Good		Fair		Poor		Don't know	All groups	
Number	61[1]	71[1]	97	92	71	66	27	21	3 —	259[2]	250[2]
Amount of treatment thought to be needed											
	Percentages										
None	57	59	47	54	28	18	7	5	≠ —	40	42
Some	41	37	46	42	61	67	44	52	≠ —	48	48
Considerable	2	1	2	1	8	11	48	38	≠ —	8	7
Don't know	—	3	4	2	3	5	—	5	≠ —	3	3
	100	100	100	100	100	100	100	100	≠ —	100	100

1. Roman figures represent Salisbury and italic figures Darlington.
2. All groups with some of their own teeth still present.
≠ Indicates numbers too small for percentage to be significant.

TABLE III.18. *Self-assessment of dental conditions analysed by amount of treatment thought to be needed*

Darlington thought they needed 'a lot' of treatment. Since the dental examiner found that 72 per cent in Salisbury, 78 per cent in Darlington of those with some teeth of their own left needed treatment for dental decay alone, these figures again show how greatly the average person underestimated the state of his or her oral health.

Attitudes towards dentistry and oral health

Subjects were asked a series of questions designed to determine the extent of their interest in oral health, and the answers to these questions may conveniently be grouped into four sections; oral hygiene and care, choice of a dentist, reaction to dental treatment, and fluoridation.

I. ORAL HYGIENE AND CARE

'Do you think that what you do now to clean and take care of your teeth (or dentures) is enough or not enough.' This was the rather challenging question put to our sample and nearly everyone thought that their oral hygiene routine was adequate. Only 10 per cent in Salisbury, 7 per cent in Darlington thought that they were not doing enough, and 2 per cent in Salisbury, 3 per cent in Darlington didn't know. Women were more complacent than men. In Salisbury 93 per cent of women compared with 82 per cent of men thought they were doing enough and in Darlington 92 per cent of women compared with 88 per cent of men. It is a pity that these answers could not have been investigated further, since four groups would probably have emerged; those who did not really believe in their answer anyway, those who gave an honest answer but had no idea of proper oral hygiene, those who gave an honest but mistaken answer, and those who gave an honest and correct answer. More information came, however, from answers to a second question, 'Do you think that what you did in the past to clean and take care of your teeth was enough or not enough?' Sixty per cent in Salisbury and 67 per cent in Darlington answered 'enough' to this question, men again being more self-critical than women. Even so, the answers show that in effect nearly two-thirds of the adults questioned considered that they had done everything possible to preserve their teeth in the past. Combining the answers to the two questions revealed that in Salisbury 56 per cent and in Darlington 63 per cent thought that they were now doing and always had done enough, and 7 per cent in Salisbury and 14 per cent in Darlington thought that they were not now doing and never had done enough to properly clean and care for their teeth.

SALISBURY

Amount of treatment thought to be needed	Sex		Age-group											Denture status			
	Males	Females	21-5	26-30	31-5	36-40	41-5	46-50	51-5	56-60	61-5	66-70	Over 70	No denture	Partial dentures	Full dentures	All groups
Number	208	257	41	28	41	52	45	49	42	45	39	26	57	146	118	201	465
	Percentages																
None	53	64	24	46	37	46	56	59	70	62	87	77	86	38	42	85	59
Some	38	27	61	39	59	39	38	33	19	29	13	20	7	48	48	10	32
Considerable	7	7	12	11	2	12	4	6	10	7	—	4	7	11	6	4	7
Don't know	1	2	2	4	2	4	2	2	2	2	—	—	—	3	3	—	2
	100	100	100	100	100	100	100	100	100	100	100	100	100	100	100	100	100

DARLINGTON

Amount of treatment thought to be needed	Sex		Age-group											Denture status			
	Males	Females	21-5	26-30	31-5	36-40	41-5	46-50	51-5	56-60	61-5	66-70	Over 70	No denture	Partial dentures	Full dentures	All groups
Number	236	280	40	44	43	52	59	55	55	46	38	29	55	183	78	255	516
	Percentages																
None	60	61	50	45	56	50	61	51	80	76	63	59	69	39	46	80	60
Some	36	32	38	50	39	42	36	46	18	22	32	28	20	51	44	18	34
Considerable	3	5	13	5	2	8	3	2	2	2	3	7	4	7	6	2	4
Don't know	2	2	—	—	2	—	—	2	—	—	3	7	7	3	4	—	2
	100	100	100	100	100	100	100	100	100	100	100	100	100	100	100	100	100

TABLE III.19. *Self-assessment of amount of dental treatment thought to be needed*

	Males		Females		Total	
Number	208[1]	236[1]	257	280	465	516
	Percentages					
Enough	82	88	93	92	88	90
Not enough	16	10	5	5	10	7
Don't know if enough	2	2	2	4	2	3
	100	100	100	100	100	100

1. Roman figures represent Salisbury and italic figures Darlington.

TABLE III.20. *Self-assessment of amount of care taken now over teeth and dentures*

	Males		Females		Total	
Number	208[1]	236[1]	257	280	465	516
	Percentages					
Enough	55	65	63	70	60	67
Not enough	44	33	35	26	39	29
Don't know if enough	1	2	2	5	1	3
	100	100	100	100	100	100

1. Roman figures represent Salisbury and italic figures Darlington.

TABLE III.21. *Self-assessment of amount of care taken in the past over teeth*

II. CHOICE OF A DENTIST

Subjects were asked, 'What do you look for in choosing a dentist?', with the aim of trying to find out why people chose the dentist they did. As already shown, people tended to stay with one dentist whether they were casual or regular attenders, so presumably familiarity played some part in subsequent visits. For the initial visit, however, the usual deciding factor quoted was the dentist's manner or personality—did he 'put you at ease'. Forty per cent of the sample in Salisbury and 30 per cent in Darlington mentioned this. Freedom from pain and recommendation by others were the next two criteria most commonly mentioned in Salisbury (35 per cent and 33 per cent) and freedom from pain was also the second factor mentioned in Darlington (27 per cent) followed by 'qualification and ability' (24 per cent), and 'recom-

	No. of people mentioning reason		Percentage of total sample	
Number	465[1]	*516*[1]		
Qualification and ability	119	*123*	26	*24*
Dentist's manner—puts you at ease	187	*153*	40	*30*
Dentist who doesn't hurt you	161	*139*	35	*27*
No waiting	60	*54*	13	*10*
Recommendation	154	*109*	33	*21*
Other reasons	140	*89*	30	*17*
Doesn't look for anything	50	*74*	11	*14*

1. Roman figures represent Salisbury and italic figures Darlington. (Percentages total more than 100 since some people mentioned more than one reason.)

TABLE III.22. *Reasons given for choice of dentist*

mendation by others' (21 per cent). Qualifications were mentioned by 26 per cent in Salisbury, followed by 'no waiting' (13 per cent) and 'don't look for anything' (11 per cent). Other factors mentioned were a dentist's ability to make a good set of dentures, or treat children, and a dentist's age—younger men being preferred as being better trained and using more modern methods.

It therefore appears that only one-quarter of the sample were interested in the qualifications or ability of their dentist. Providing he had a winning personality and did not inflict any pain this seemed to be as far as most people looked in their choice, especially women. Men looked more for short waiting times and relied more on the recommendation of others. Surprisingly, hardly anyone mentioned accessibility, which suggested that many people might merely go to their nearest dentist, rather than actually choosing one.

Qualifications and manner were mentioned more often in the non-manual groups, and lack of waiting time and freedom from pain by the manual groups. Recommendations were mentioned more often by full denture wearers, especially in Salisbury.

III. REACTION TO DENTAL TREATMENT

'Are you nervous when you go to the dentist?' Surprisingly, the answers were not 100 per cent 'yes' but only 35 per cent 'yes' in

	Males		Females		Total	
Number	207[1]	232[1]	256	279	463[2]	511[2]
	Percentages					
Nervous	26	20	44	42	35	32
Not nervous	74	80	55	58	63	68
Don't know if nervous	—	—	1	—	1	—
	100	100	100	100	100	100

1. Roman figures represent Salisbury and italic figures Darlington.
2. Two persons in Salisbury and five in Darlington who told us they had never been to the dentist were not asked this question.

TABLE III.23. *If nervous when visiting dentist*

Salisbury and 32 per cent 'yes' in Darlington. It must be remembered though that nearly half of those asked were full denture wearers with little further to fear from a dentist other than the possible unpleasantness of taking denture impressions. In fact only 27 per cent in Salisbury, and 24 per cent in Darlington of the full denture wearers answered 'yes', leaving about 40 per cent of those with their own teeth also admitting to being nervous. Not surprisingly, fewer men than women confessed to being nervous, although men are far more likely to faint in a dentist's chair than women! Younger people tended to be more nervous than older people, and fear clearly emerged as a factor keeping people away from the dentist. Fewer regular attenders were nervous than occasional or 'pain only' attenders.

	Males		Females		Total	
Number	53[1]	46[1]	112	116	165	162
	Percentages					
Treatment	21	35	29	38	26	37
Waiting	6	—	4	4	4	3
Everything	49	48	58	39	55	41
Other reasons / Don't know why / nervous	25	22	17	22	19	22

1. Roman figures represent Salisbury and italic figures Darlington.
(Percentages total more than 100 since some people mentioned more than one reason.)

TABLE III.24. *Reasons given for being nervous about visiting the dentist*

Those who answered 'yes' to the last question were asked what particularly made them nervous, and about half mentioned in reply some aspect of treatment—'the drill' or 'pain'. Twenty-six per cent in Salisbury, 37 per cent in Darlington said that everything about going to a dentist scared them, but about 4 per cent in both areas said that it was only the waiting that worried them—once in the chair they were all right. About 20 per cent gave other reasons for their nervousness or did not know why they were nervous. It was not only the treatment, therefore, that worried people, but also waiting for it.

Another aspect of dental treatment is its cost. Was the average person satisfied with N.H.S. charges for dental treatment? Most people, 63 per cent in Salisbury, 68 per cent in Darlington were satisfied, but 17 per cent in Salisbury, 22 per cent in Darlington thought the charges were too high generally, and a further 8 per cent in Salisbury, 5 per cent in Darlington thought that at least some of the charges were too high. Eleven per cent in Salisbury, 5 per cent in Darlington said that they did not know what the N.H.S. charges were. This last group was met with most frequently among the under-25s. Greatest satisfaction with N.H.S. charges occurred in the 35–60 age-groups, but manual workers were less satisfied than non-manual workers. The highest numbers dissatisfied with N.H.S. charges were found among those who had only visited a dentist when in pain; 1 in every 4 in Salisbury and 1 in every 3 in Darlington. Perhaps surprisingly, about one-

	Number		Percentage	
Satisfactory	221[1]	*252*[1]	63	*68*
Middling—some satisfactory,				
some high	29	*19*	8	*5*
High	60	*81*	17	*22*
Not known	38	*20*	11	*5*
	348	*372*	100	*100*

1. Roman figures represent Salisbury and italic figures Darlington.

TABLE III.25. *Attitudes of N.H.S. dental patients to charges for N.H.S. dental treatment*

eighth of the self-styled 'regular' attenders did not know what the
N.H.S. charges were! More full denture wearers than others were
satisfied with the N.H.S. cost of treatment, and conversely fewer
non-denture wearers were content with it.

The attitude of private patients towards their treatment has
already been mentioned (p. 41). N.H.S. patients were asked for
their opinions on both private treatment and private service; how
did they think it compared with their own service and treatment?
Only 18 per cent in Salisbury and 15 per cent in Darlington
thought that private treatment would be better than N.H.S.
treatment, the percentage being slightly higher in the younger
age-groups. However, in Salisbury nearly 30 per cent of Classes
I and II thought that private treatment would be better, although
fewer than average thought so in Classes III non-manual and V.
Social class differences were less marked in Darlington, although
the trend there was the reverse of that found in Salisbury. Apart
from treatment, 22 per cent in Salisbury, 12 per cent in Darlington
thought they would get better service from a private dentist, and
in both towns 85 per cent rated treatment and service equally,
making no distinctions between the two. When asked why they
thought private treatment would be better, reasons given included
more attention given to saving teeth and fitting dentures. Reasons
for better private service included less waiting for an appointment
and in the waiting room.

IV. ATTITUDES TOWARDS FLUORIDATION

Fluoridation of public water supplies is a dental health measure
which has aroused strong feelings and resulted in considerable
publicity, with ardent advocates and opponents. At the time of
the survey, fluoridation had been more often a topic for public and
political discussion in Darlington than in Salisbury where it had
appeared more as an indirect national than as a direct local issue.
Two aspects of this matter seemed to be important in terms of
attitudes to oral health. Firstly, how many people knew what
fluoridation was about, and secondly, of those who had some idea
about it, how many approved or disapproved of it? Here was a
means of judging not only the average person's interest in oral

	Number		Percentage of total		Percentage of those who have heard of fluoridation	
Approve	143[1]	*136*[1]	31	*26*	46	*32*
Disapprove	21	*105*	5	*29*	7	*25*
Undecided	144	*186*	31	*36*	47	*44*
Never heard of fluoridation⎫ Did not know what fluori- ⎬ dation was ⎭	157	*89*	34	*17*	—	—
	465	*516*	100	*100*	100	*100*

1. Roman figures represent Salisbury and italic figures Darlington.

TABLE III.26. *Attitudes towards fluoridation*

health matters but also his reaction to a measure which could affect him personally.

In Salisbury 34 per cent of the adult sample had never heard of fluoridation, compared with only 17 per cent in Darlington. Considering now only those who had a correct idea of what is involved in fluoridation, 7 per cent in Salisbury and 25 per cent in Darlington disapproved of it. Forty-six per cent in Salisbury and 32 per cent in Darlington approved of it and 47 per cent in Salisbury, 44 per cent in Darlington were undecided. Of the total sample, 5 per cent in Salisbury and 29 per cent in Darlington disapproved of fluoridation. It should be mentioned here that in Darlington the issue had become closely related to party politics, and to some degree opinion was probably less the result of personal conviction than the following of a party line. Incidentally, many people confused fluoridation with chlorination; a pitfall first discovered on the pilot survey. Somewhat fewer women than men in both areas understood fluoridation, but parents of children under ten were better informed than others. Non-manual workers were more likely to have heard about fluoridation than manual workers, 23 per cent in Salisbury and 7 per cent in Darlington of the non-manual groups had not heard of fluoridation, compared with 40 per cent in Salisbury, 21 per cent in Darlington of the manual workers. Most of those ignorant of fluoridation were irregular dental attenders, and in the older age-groups.

Attitude to fluoridation	Reason given for attitude	No. in group		Percentage of group mentioning reason	
Approve:	Prevents decay			12	*11*
	Helps children's teeth	143[1]	*136[1]*	41	*34*
	Does good			23	*42*
	Other reasons			26	*13*
Disapprove:	Mass medication			10	*13*
	Leave water alone	21	*105*	62	*32*
	Harmful effects			24	*21*
	Other reasons			33	*28*
Undecided:	Two sides to issue			69	*45*
	Don't care	144	*186*	13	*15*
	Not thought about it			19	*41*

1. Roman figures represent Salisbury and italic figures Darlington. (Percentages total more than 100 since some respondents gave more than one reason.)

TABLE III.27. *Reasons given for attitude to fluoridation*

Of those who were undecided about their reaction to fluoridation, 13 per cent in Salisbury and 15 per cent in Darlington said that it did not matter to them if fluoride were added to drinking water or not. These were mainly older people. Most of the 'undecided' group, however, thought that there were two sides to the question and they did not know which was right. Many also thought the over-all cost too high when only young children would benefit. Another small group thought that no matter how beneficial the results, it was wrong to treat compulsorily everybody's water supplies.

Of those favouring fluoridation, 41 per cent in Salisbury, 34 per cent in Darlington, said it 'helped children's teeth', and 23 per cent in Salisbury and 42 per cent in Darlington said that it 'did good'. Only 21 people disapproved of fluoridation in Salisbury, and of these 13 said that the water should be kept 'pure' and left alone. Twenty-one per cent in Darlington mentioned a possibly harmful effect of fluoride on the body.

To sum up, those in favour of fluoridation were found mainly among men, younger people, non-manual and skilled manual workers, those without dentures, and 'regular' dental attenders.

IV *Discussion*

This Report has so far presented data obtained during the course of the investigation without considering in any detail its less obvious implications with reference to the original questions on dental attitudes and dental need and demand which initiated the work. An attempt is now made to remedy this.

National relevance

The two areas chosen for the investigation differed in many ways, as detailed earlier, yet in spite of this the results of many lines of inquiry were found to be similar in both towns. It would therefore be easy to assume that these data could apply equally well to other parts of the country or even to the country as a whole. There is, however, no evidence whatsoever either to confirm or to deny this assumption, and points of similarity may well be simple coincidences. The data must therefore be considered to apply only to the two areas in question, and national implications must wait on national surveys.

Sample reliability

Evidence has already been presented on the representative nature of the two sample populations and the biases introduced by interview and examination refusals and 'non-contacts'. The main subdivisions of the samples have been by age, sex, and social class based on the type of occupation followed by the heads of households. There has been much argument among sociologists about

E

both the concept of social class and the criteria by which it can be recognized. Occupations have been used as the criteria here partly because of ease of comparison with Census data and other studies and partly because no better criteria presented themselves.

One further point. The pattern of dental disease and treatment is such that inevitably data in some categories must be based on a small number of individuals. For example, hardly anyone over the age of 65 can be expected to have more than a few of their own teeth left. Data on teeth present in these cases cannot therefore be as numerous as that from the younger age-groups. The condition of teeth in the aged population, if it is to be fully studied, needs special sampling techniques inappropriate to this survey. Where relevant this has been taken into account when presenting data both in the earlier sections and in this discussion.

In order to be able to present an accurate picture of a community's oral health and attitudes towards oral health three lines of investigation are necessary. These are investigations into (1) treatment needed, (2) treatment sought, and (3) treatment provided. Each of these will now be considered in turn.

Dental treatment needed

Evidence concerning the need for dental treatment has been provided by the data obtained from the dental examinations. In common with many other forms of medical treatment, however, there is rarely one specific treatment for a specific disease problem. Consider for example a decayed tooth: the accepted ideal treatment for this, since the decay process is irreversible, is to remove the affected tooth substance and restore the tooth contour with a filling material such as silver amalgam or gold. But if the tooth were badly decayed or in a chronically neglected mouth the preferred treatment might well be extraction since the chances of successful permanent restoration would be remote. In other words it is necessary to consider the individual case before coming to any general conclusions on dental treatment. Ten decayed teeth do not necessarily indicate the need for ten restorations. This complicates the reporting of treatment needs since one of the suitable methods would be to report in terms of chairside hours of work required; yet whether a given tooth needs a one-hour gold inlay or a ten-minute extraction lies entirely at the discretion of the individual dentist concerned. Of course, working times vary considerably between one dentist and another, so that only 'average' times can be used. These observations must be borne in mind when the following estimates of treatment needs in the two survey areas are considered. These estimates are based on treatment plans made out by the dental examiner from the dental examination results of a randomly selected 20 per cent of all subjects examined, and converted into chairside hours of work from a table of timings for individual operations obtained after consultation with colleagues in specialized and general dental practice. They are therefore intended merely to indicate the magnitude of this problem of treatment need. It was estimated that the average Salisbury adult needed a little more than $1\frac{1}{2}$ hours of chairside dental treatment, and the average Darlington adult about $1\frac{1}{4}$ hours of chairside treatment. Put another way, about 60 dentists working a 35-hour chairside week for 6 months would be needed to bring the adult population of Salisbury to a state of dental fitness, and 90 dentists working for the same time in Darlington. Individuals in Darlington tended to need less work than individuals in Salisbury simply because they tended to have fewer saveable teeth and more satisfactory full dentures.

A further factor to be considered when dealing with treatment needs is the difference between 'initial' and 'maintenance' dental care. Initial care is the work required to bring a person to a state of sound dental health, and maintenance care is as its name suggests the routine treatment then required at intervals to maintain him or her in that state. Data on this difference are lacking in this country, but work in the United States suggests that initial care there probably takes about three times the chairside time required for maintenance care per annum.[1] It is therefore probably less time-consuming for a dentist to be able to maintain a person in a state of sound oral health than to have to restore to

1. Young, W. O., and Striffler, F. S., *The Dentist, his Practice and the Community* (Saunders. Philadelphia. 1964).

health a neglected mouth. This logically leads on to a discussion of the demand for dental treatment or 'treatment sought', but before embarking on this, one final matter remains to be considered under the heading of 'treatment needed'. Briefly, then, 'Why is dental treatment needed?' Why not, indeed, have all teeth extracted at some early and convenient time in life and then wear full dentures. By doing this the possible agonies of toothache are avoided and also the routine periods of discomfort in a dentist's chair with even then very little hope of retaining natural teeth to any great age, especially as life-expectancy becomes longer. This argument was frequently met with during the course of the survey, and requires a reasonable answer. Probably the best answer is to observe that so far no denture has been devised which can begin to approach the efficiency and comfort of natural teeth. The full denture wearer will in time become accustomed to his dentures and even cease to be aware of them, but at first they are two foreign bodies in his mouth which require the mastery of completely new masticatory techniques if they are to function with any efficiency. Not everyone, indeed, ever achieves this mastery. The problem of dentures and attitudes towards dentures will be considered later, and it is sufficient to say in this context that our data indicate that professed satisfaction with a set of dentures bears little relation to the actual efficiency of those dentures.

Dental treatment sought

Information on the demand for dental treatment comes almost exclusively from a study of the attitudes of the individual towards dentistry and oral health. Two factors are involved, firstly awareness of oral health problems and secondly willingness to seek dental examination and treatment. These two factors may be considered separately.

Oral health awareness

If a disease is symptomless in the early stages, that is, if the victim is unaware of anything wrong, treatment may become impossible simply because the victim did not present himself for treatment in time. If, however, the potential victim knows that the disease is symptomless in the early stages, he may be more inclined to seek a medical examination as a matter of routine and the disease may be stopped in its early stages. So it is with oral disease. Many people sincerely believe that a dentist is someone to be visited only when they have toothache, by which time, of course, the offending tooth may be unsaveable and have to be extracted. Thus, to them, a dentist is someone who takes teeth out more or less painfully and therefore is someone to be avoided except in cases of emergency. They do not appreciate, because they have never understood, that dental or periodontal disease starts long before toothache. A second group of people are aware of the need for regular dental check-ups even though they may not know the reason for the need, but they still do not attend either from fear or because oral health has a low priority in their way of life. Long waiting-lists and inconvenient appointment times will, of course, also affect their decision.

A third and final group is of those who attend their dentist regularly. Our data show that only 20 per cent of the sample interviewed in Salisbury and 10 per cent in Darlington claimed to be in the third group, although a further 10 per cent in both towns said that their last visit had been a routine check-up. Therefore at least 70 per cent of the sample in Salisbury and 80 per cent of the sample in Darlington fell into the first two groups, and the question must be asked 'Are people being sufficiently educated in oral health matters?' Care must be taken here in defining oral health education and its possible results. It is not suggested that a 100 per cent effective oral health education scheme would result in 100 per cent regular attendance for dental treatment. There will always be a substantial group of people who even though they are aware of the problem will give it a low priority in their way of life or be fearful at the thought of treatment. This has been shown to be the case in far more serious conditions than oral disease. A fully effective oral health education system would not, therefore, eliminate the second group of people mentioned above, but it would eliminate the first group. In other words, far more people would be aware of the problem and be free to make their own decision about the action they should take, rather than, as at the moment, a substantial group being unaware of the existence of any problem at all.

What form should this oral health education take? Data from the two areas suggest that at present oral health education is having little effect on the people at whom it is aimed. The main message being put across seems to be 'Clean your teeth regularly, don't eat sweets between meals, visit your dentist regularly and your teeth will never be any trouble to you. Fail in any of these rules and you will suffer from toothache.' The trouble with this is that it is too dogmatic and so becomes illogical. We probably all know people who follow the rules but still suffer from tooth-ache and others who do not follow the rules and yet rarely have dental trouble. The result is that while the average person may be well aware of these rules for good oral health he or she does not follow them because he sees no logic in them. 'I've always cleaned my teeth regularly and visited my dentist regularly and for all the good it's done I might just as well not have bothered', said one Salisbury lady to us and the same theme recurred at frequent intervals throughout the survey. A shift of emphasis to cause rather than remedy seems to be needed to bring the case for proper oral care home to people. This in turn requires more than talks from dentists and ancillary workers or the odd 'dental health campaign' of varying duration. More important seems to be the need for dental health education as part of a regular course of personal hygiene in schools, as is already taught in many countries and as is being planned by some education authorities in this country. All secondary schoolchildren should be at least made aware of the origins and pattern of dental and periodontal disease and how these diseases may best be limited or prevented. They should be taught to look upon dirty and badly cared for teeth as being as socially unacceptable as dirty hair, nails, feet, or bodies. Until such education is effective, dentists will continue to spend much of their time extracting stumps from mouths ruined by neglect and finally providing full dentures when the battle is ultimately lost.

The advantages of such a system of health education would be twofold. In the first place it is probable, although not inevitable, that more people would become regular rather than emergency dental attenders; and in the second place dentists would be able to discuss their patients' cases with them and be able to rely far more upon their co-operation—a factor vital to successful sustained dental treatment and the avoidance of wasted treatment. This theme is developed further in the following section on readiness to attend for dental treatment, and we close this section with the observation that it is a sad commentary on the state of dental knowledge in this country when it is found that an intelligent professional man here apparently knows less about oral health than a 9-year-old schoolgirl in California. It is significant in this context to note that if the same Californian schoolgirl attended a school dental inspection with dirty teeth she would in all probability be sent home with a request for a parental explanation.

Willingness to attend for treatment or examination

Our data show that people are still deterred from visiting a dentist through fear that they will be hurt and tend to go to a dentist with a reputation for 'gentleness', a quality put before any other when choosing a dentist. While freedom from pain during treatment should be the aim of all dentists, it is inevitable that some dental procedures will be uncomfortable and a few even briefly painful. It would be wrong to minimize this, and it would perhaps be better if patients understood why some procedures were likely to be more distressing than others than for them to be faced with an over-all fear of the unknown. 'I wouldn't mind it hurting so much if I knew when it was going to', we were told more than once. This is partly a matter of dental education and partly a matter of regular attendance from an early age to breed familiarity with dental procedures. As mentioned earlier in another context, someone attending a dentist as an emergency case with raging toothache is not likely to receive painless treatment since even touching the offending tooth may be exquisitely painful.

After fear, time seems to be an important factor in determining regular dental attendance. This is particularly true in the case of manual workers who probably not only stand to lose more money by visiting a dentist than non-manual workers but may also have more difficulty in obtaining leave from work, although there is admittedly little evidence to support this latter surmise. It is, however, frequently difficult if not impossible for people, including children, to obtain leave of absence from work or school in order to visit a dentist for a course of treatment during normal working hours. The late hours worked by many dentists bear witness to this. If, let us suppose, there was a statutory obligation on all employers and head teachers to allow their employees or pupils two paid 'dental leave' sessions per year it would be interesting to see if the number of regular attenders increased and the number of emergencies decreased, and if the total working hours lost through workers having to seek emergency treatment decreased.

In this country the cost of dental treatment is not a very significant factor since anyone may obtain subsidized treatment through the N.H.S. It is interesting, however, that in both areas over a quarter of the samples interviewed thought that at least some of the present N.H.S. dental charges were too high, and that where an expensive item such as dentures was involved, a higher proportion of people sought N.H.S. rather than private treatment than was the case with other less expensive types of treatment. Private treatment was apparently received by little more than 10 per cent of the sample in Salisbury and a somewhat higher percentage in Darlington—the private patients giving reasons of better service and better treatment for their choice. A significant number of these were manual workers receiving emergency treatment and it could well be that being paid by the hour they lost less money by paying more for rapid treatment than by paying less for treatment involving a considerable wait.

Summarizing the question of dental demand, it is first of all clear that at the moment demand for treatment is nowhere near so great as the need for dental treatment in the two survey areas. This appears to be due primarily to ignorance of the nature of oral disease and the advantages to be obtained by regular treatment and secondarily to fear of the dentist and reluctance to be put to the trouble of regular visits especially when these involve considerable waiting time both for an appointment and in the waiting-room. This in turn relates to the number of dentists available to provide treatment. The dentist is still looked upon by too many people as an extractor of teeth and a provider of full dentures. Admittedly this attitude was more common in Darlington than in Salisbury, but although more conservative treatment was apparent in Salisbury, there was little more understanding there of the logic of restorations as opposed to extractions. 'He said he'd fill them so I told him to go ahead and do what he liked. I didn't mind!' While this attitude is better than that of the patient who insists that he knows more than his dentist about his treatment needs ('I told him fillings weren't any good—I told him to take them out'), it still falls far short of the ideal of a patient understanding what his dentist is doing and appreciating the final result. Finally, to too many people a good dentist is one who does not hurt them and a bad dentist is one who does—irrespective of the quality of work produced.

Treatment provided

The final section of this survey of community oral health will be dealt with quite briefly as in the main it falls outside our terms of reference. The biggest treatment difference between the two communities was the higher proportion of full dentures seen in Darlington and the higher proportion of restored teeth seen in Salisbury. In other words, people in Darlington tended to have teeth extracted rather than filled to a greater extent than in Salisbury. This was to be expected if only because of the different dentist/population ratios and it is interesting that so far as it is possible to judge, the conservative output per dentist was the same in both areas, that is, the number of fillings per dentist was the same in each area. Given a more favourable dentist/population ratio in Darlington it is, however, still impossible to say whether a greater proportion of the population would then prefer restorations to extractions or if the proportions would become similar to those obtained in Salisbury.

It would be wrong to close this section without commenting on the amount of neglected or wasted treatment seen in both areas. By this is meant restored teeth which have been allowed to become grossly re-decayed due to neglect, or dentures which no longer fit through age or which are cracked or broken. The probable reasons for this have been discussed in previous sections, and the special problems of denture wearers are discussed in the next section, which is devoted entirely to them since they constitute over half the adult population.

Denture wearers

One of our most surprising findings was the high proportion of dentures being worn which for one reason or another were considered on examination to be less than satisfactory. These made up nearly half the total number of full dentures seen in Darlington and about two-thirds of those seen in Salisbury. Yet questioning showed that most of the owners of these dentures were perfectly happy with them, or if they did have any complaints they did not consider them sufficiently important to take any action to remedy them. Cracked dentures, dentures with teeth and flanges missing, unmatched pairs of dentures, and dentures which fitted so badly that they had caused tissue damage or else were retained only by the skill and caution of the wearer's long experience—all these were being worn regularly. Frequently too, poorly fitting dentures were being worn in preference to newer, better-fitting sets, especially by elderly people. In fact the chances of a new denture being tolerated by an elderly person whose old set had been worn for 10 or 15 years were poor. The longer a denture was worn the more it was tolerated no matter how badly it came to fit or how damaged it became. This leads to the alarming thought that in all probability badly fitting dentures in the first instance would come to be accepted by the average denture wearer just as readily as properly fitting dentures.

Most denture wearers clearly had no idea that dentures need

to be checked at regular intervals if they are to retain their efficiency. Certainly very few ever bothered to have their dentures checked as the attendance figures for both areas show. Criticism of dentures seemed to be most frequent at the newly edentulous stage, tailing off rapidly until it became non-existent even though merited. It is significant that when asked if they had trouble eating, over three-quarters of the full denture wearers said that they never did; a similar proportion to those non-denture wearers giving the same answer. This cannot be taken as indicating that denture and non-denture wearers eat the same things with the same ease. Indeed far more than one-quarter of the full dentures seen were quite obviously useless for such normal masticatory purposes as chewing a toffee or biting into an apple. The full denture wearers were presumably indicating that within their self-imposed dietary restrictions they experienced no trouble in eating; this is a point worthy of closer investigation, since it is difficult to reconcile the actual state of our samples' dentures with their own feelings concerning them. It could, of course, be argued that the inability to chew toffee or meat or bite into apples can hardly be regarded as a hardship. Even if this is true, however, it still does not alter the fact that eating habits must inevitably change after the acquisition of full dentures, and that the extent of this change is a measure of the failure of the dentures to replace the natural dentition.

Our sociological data show interesting differences in attitude between non-denture wearers in the two survey areas concerning the prospect of one day having to wear dentures. In Salisbury, for example, where fewer adults wore full dentures, 28 per cent of the non-denture wearers both expected to have to wear dentures eventually and were not bothered by this thought, whereas in Darlington, where a higher proportion wore full dentures, only 20 per cent of the non-denture wearers were equally serene. In Salisbury only 23 per cent of the non-denture wearers hoped that they would not need dentures compared with 54 per cent in Darlington. Darlington, therefore, the area with proportionally more full dentures and those proportionally better maintained than in Salisbury was also the area where more non-denture wearers were apprehensive at the thought of wearing dentures. This is an unexpected finding and therefore not easy to explain. To suggest that in Darlington the disadvantages of full dentures are more obvious because there are more full dentures being worn is to come to an unjustifiable conclusion. Possibly this is a difference in area temperament. Salisbury tends to be less decisive, more dentally apathetic than Darlington as exemplified by the higher proportion of unsatisfactory dentures being worn and tolerated there. It could be argued that in the same way the thought of having to wear dentures eventually was 'tolerated' without too much anxiety in Salisbury. In Darlington on the other hand there was less tolerance of bad dentures and a more realistic approach to the thought of having to wear dentures. In this connection it is also significant that only 10 per cent of the non-denture wearers in Darlington did not expect to have to wear dentures, compared with 16 per cent in Salisbury.

Conclusion

What, briefly, did the survey achieve? In conclusion we attempt to answer this question in tabular form.

GENERAL

1. It was demonstrated that a survey of this nature was not only practically possible but would meet with a sufficiently cooperative response to achieve significant results.

2. Area differences in the pattern of oral health were shown to exist both in terms of actual oral state and in attitudes towards oral health.

DENTAL

3. About three-quarters of the adult population samples including full-denture wearers were shown to be in need of dental treatment. Over 90 per cent of non-denture wearers needed treatment of one kind or another.

4. In Salisbury 42 per cent and in Darlington 51 per cent of the adult sample were shown to have no natural teeth left at all; the average number of teeth present per adult being 12 in Salisbury and 10 in Darlington.

5. Approximately three-quarters of all adults with teeth of their own were found to have decayed teeth.

6. Approximately 70 per cent of the adult sample in both towns were shown to require periodontal treatment.

SOCIO-DENTAL

7. The need for dental treatment was shown to exceed greatly the demand for such treatment, both in denture and non-denture wearers.

8. Lay self-assessments of oral health in general or in detail were shown to bear little relation to the actual oral state, and the criteria used in arriving at these self-assessments were shown to bear no relation to those used by a dentist.

9. Most of the adult sample were shown to be unaware of the existence of periodontal disease.

10. Oral health awareness was shown to be rarely met with in a practical as opposed to a theoretical sense. The rules were known but not practised.

11. A considerable amount of dental treatment was subsequently wasted due to ignorance and hence neglect.

SOCIOLOGICAL

12. Dental visiting patterns were shown to vary considerably according to age and social status.

13. Only 1 adult in 5 in Salisbury and 1 adult in 10 in Darlington claimed to have visited a dentist regularly during the previous 5 years.

14. Only 10 per cent of the sample claimed that they received private dental treatment.

15. Sixty per cent of the samples thought they required no dental treatment, and 40 per cent of those not wearing full dentures.

16. Approximately 90 per cent in both areas thought they were doing enough to clean and care for their teeth or dentures, but only 60–70 per cent thought they had done enough in the past.

17. Dentists were shown to be chosen mainly by their supposed 'gentleness' and ease of manner. Rapid treatment with little waiting about was important to manual workers.

18. Only one-third of the sample claimed to be nervous when visiting a dentist, although this included 40 per cent of the non-denture wearers.

19. Over one-quarter of the samples thought the cost of N.H.S. dentistry was too high in general or in particular.

20. Thirty-four per cent in Salisbury and 17 per cent in Darlington had never heard of fluoridation. Of those who understood it, only 7 per cent in Salisbury and 25 per cent in Darlington disapproved of it. (It had been a 'political' issue in Darlington.)

This survey has been in all respects a pilot. The information obtained has paved the way for, and shown the need of, a more searching national survey on dental needs and dental attitudes.

Our thanks are due to those people in Salisbury and Darlington who so generously and patiently helped us with our work. Without their frequently enthusiastic help this survey would have been doomed to failure. It is with pleasure that we recall the time spent among them.

Appendices

Appendix A. *Questionnaire*

PERSONAL DATA (SUBJECT)

Name ....Age ....
Address ....
....
District

Interviewer ....
Date of interview ....
Time started .... ended ....
Time taken for interview .... minutes ....
Other persons present at interview ....
....
....

F

Interviewer's comments

....

Best times for dental examination ....

Telephone ....

SQ1

A. GENERAL

1. Would you say that your general health is:

   Good 1
   Fair 2
   Poor 3
   D.K. 4

2. How much trouble have teeth and gums been to you throughout life?

   If 'a lot' or 'some trouble'
   What sort of trouble?

   ....

   A lot of trouble...... 5
   Some trouble......... 6
   Little trouble 7
   No trouble............ 8
   D.K. 9

3. About how many of your permanent teeth have you lost?

   If 'some' or 'all' lost
   (a) Were any of these lost for reasons other than decay?

   ....

   None 1
   Some (specify) 2
   All 3
   D.K. 4
   Yes (specify) 5
   No 6
   D.K. 7

(b) Do you perhaps *have* some form of denture? (removable false teeth or tooth)

Yes 1
No 2
                  N.D.
D.K. 3
Full upper and lower 4
                  F.D.
Partial 5
                  P.D

If 'yes'
What type of denture?

4. **Ask all except 'full denture'**
   (a) What state do you think your *own* teeth are in now?

Very good 1
Good 2
Fair 3
Poor 4
D.K. 5

   (b) Are there ways in which you would like your teeth to be better?
   ....

Yes (specify) 6
No 7
D.K. 8

5. How would you describe the state of your gums? Are they:
   If 'fair' or 'poor'
   What then is the trouble?
   ....

Healthy 1
Fair 2
Poor 3
D.K. 4

6. How often do teeth or dentures cause you trouble when eating?

Often 5
Sometimes 6
Never 7
D.K. 8

7. Have you heard of fluoridation of water supplies?

Yes 1
No 2
D.K. 3

   If 'yes'
   How do you feel about fluoridation of water supplies?
   Probe all answers
   Why do you say this?
   ....

Do you approve ... 4
Do you disapprove 5
Are you undecided 6

B. NOW SOME QUESTIONS ABOUT VISITING THE DENTIST

8. Have your teeth ever been *examined* by a dentist?

    If 'no' or 'D.K.'—probe:
    Not even at school, in the Forces, in a hospital (or—*if applicable*—in a maternity clinic)?
    If 'no' or 'D.K.' go on to Qu. 40

    Yes 1
    No 2
    D.K./can't remember 3

9. Roughly how old were you when your teeth were first *examined* by a dentist?
    If remember teeth seen before age 15 or before leaving school
    What do you particularly remember about early childhood visits to the dentist?

    .... years old
    D.K.   ....

    D.K.   ....

    ....

10. Can you say something about visits to the dentist since childhood—about how often you went, and anything you specially remember?

Age	Visits to dentist						Special comments
Record age now: ☐ years	once a year or more often	occasional (less than once a year)	only if in pain	only for work on dentures	none	D.K./ Can't remember	
First visits −14	1	2	3	4	5	6	
15–29	1	2	3	4	5	6	
30–44	1	2	3	4	5	6	
45–	1	2	3	4	5	6	
In last five years	1	2	3	4	5	6	

11. Has anything ever prevented you from going to a dentist when you thought you should have gone?

Yes (specify) 1
No 2
D.K. 3

....

12. When was your *last visit* to the dentist? **If within the last 12 months probe carefully and record month if known**

...... month ...... year
.... months ago
.... years ago
D.K. ....

If last visit more than 5 years ago or 'D.K.'—go on to Qu. 23

Questions 13–22 for visits within the last five years

13. Why did you go for your last series of visits?

....

14. (*a*) Can you also remember when you went for your *previous series* of visits? **If within the last 12 months probe carefully and record month if known** **Ask all except 'full denture'**

...... month ...... year
.... months ago
.... years ago
D.K. ....

(*b*) When do you expect your *next visit* will be?

...... months from now
...... years from now
D.K. ....

(*c*) Have you an appointment fixed now?

Yes 1
No 2
D.K. 3

15. Have you a regular dentist? **If 'yes'** How did you come to go to this particular dentist/practice?

Yes (regular dentist) 1
Yes (regular practice) 2
No 3
D.K. 4

....

16. In which town does your regular dentist (the last dentist you saw) practise? **If not survey town** Why do you have your treatment in (name town)?

....
town

....

17. (*a*) Are you nervous when you go to the dentist?   Yes 1
                                                                No 2
     If 'yes'   D.K. 3
     What about?

     ....

     (*b*) Do you feel about the same, better, or worse than in past visits to the dentist?   About the same...... 4
                             Better 5
                             Worse................... 6
     If 'better' or 'worse'   No previous visit ... 7
     Why is this?   D.K. 8

     ....

18. Is there perhaps something about your dentist, his staff, surgery, or waiting room, that you particularly like?
     Dentist: Staff:
     Surgery: Waiting-room:

19. Is there perhaps also something about dentists, their staff, surgeries or waiting rooms, that you don't like so much?
     Dentists: Staff:
     Surgeries: Waiting-rooms:

20. (*a*) In about the last *five years* did you need to go to the dentist for *emergency* treatment?   Yes 1
                             No 2
                             D.K. 3
     (*b*) During this time have you failed to get in to see a dentist?   Yes 4
                             No 5
     If 'yes'   D.K. 6
     How was that?

     ....

21. Have you ever changed your dentist?   Yes 1
     If 'yes'   Yes (same practice) 2
     What was the reason for the *last change*?   No 3
     ....   D.K. 4

22. How satisfied have you been with the dental treatment you have had in about the *last five years*?   Very satisfied 5
                             Fairly satisfied 6
                             Not really satisfied... 7
     If 'fairly' or 'not really satisfied'   D.K. 8
     Why was this?

     ....

     Now go on to Qu. 30

Questions 23–9 for visits more than 5 years ago (Look back to Qu. 12)

Last visit:

☐ years ago

23. What do you remember about your *last series* of visits?

....

D.K. when............

D.K. ....

24. Since the last visit have you had any dental trouble?
    If 'yes'
    (*a*) What was it?

....

(*b*) Why then didn't you go to a dentist?

....

Yes 1
No 2
D.K. 3

25. **Ask all except 'full denture'**
    When do you expect your *next visit* will be?

...... months from now
...... years from now
D.K.

26. Were you nervous when you went for your *last series* of visits?
    If 'yes'
    What about?

....

Yes 1
No 2
D.K. 3

27. Was there perhaps something about the last dentist you saw, his staff, surgery, or waiting room, that you particularly liked?

Dentist: Staff:
Surgery: Waiting-room:

28. Is there perhaps also something about dentists, their staff, surgeries, or waiting rooms, that you don't like so much?
    Dentists: Staff:
    Surgeries: Waiting-rooms:

29. How satisfied were you with your *last series* of dental treatment?
    If 'fairly' or 'not really satisfied'
    Why was this?

....

Very satisfied   1
Fairly satisfied   2
Not really satisfied... 3
D.K. 4

C. NOW SOME QUESTIONS ABOUT DENTURES

Check denture status—look back to   No dentures ... N.D.
Qu. 3b   Dentures ...P.D....F.D.

If no dentures—ask 30, 31   If has dentures—ask 32–4

For those with no dentures:

30. Does the thought of wearing dentures   Yes 1
    bother you?   No 2
    If 'yes' or 'no'   D.K. 3
    Why do you think this?

    ....

31. Do you think in fact you will ever need   Yes 4
    dentures?   Hope not 5
                                                  No 6
    Now go on to Qu. 35   D.K. 7

For those with dentures

32. About how long have you had some   .... months
    form of denture?   .... years
                                                      D.K.

33. Have you any complaints about your   Yes 1
    dentures?   No 2
    If 'yes'   D.K. 3
    (*a*) What type of denture is it?   Full upper and lower 4
    (*b*) What complaints?   Full upper... 5
                                             Full lower 6
    ....
    (*c*) Have you tried to do anything about   Partial 7
    it? ....

34. Do you now wish that you had kept your   Yes 8
    own teeth?   No 9
    If 'yes' or 'no'   D.K. 10
    Why is this?

    ....

D. NOW SOME QUESTIONS ABOUT TREATMENT UNDER THE N.H.S.

35. Do you usually have your treatment under the N.H.S., or do you pay for it privately?

    N.H.S. 1
    Private 2
    Not been since 1948 3
    D.K. 4

    (*A form is signed in treatment under the N.H.S.*)

    **If 'N.H.S.'—ask 36, 37   If 'private'—ask 38, 39
    If 'not been since 1948' or 'D.K.'—go to 44
    If N.H.S.:**

36. If you paid for all your dental work *privately*, would you expect (*a*) the treatment, (*b*) the service, to be about the same, better or worse, than under N.H.S.?

	About same	Better	Worse	D.K.
Treatment	... 1	... 2	... 3	... 4
Service	... 5	... 6	... 7	... 8

    If 'better'
    In what way better?
    ....

37. **Ask only those over 21**
    What do you think of the charges for dental treatment under N.H.S.?
    ....

    Now go on to Qu. 44

    If private:
38. For what reasons do you choose privately paid dental treatment?
    ....

39. Have you ever had any dental treatment under the N.H.S.?

    Yes 1
    No 2

    Now go on to Qu. 44

    D.K. 3

E. IF TEETH NEVER EXAMINED BY A DENTIST

40. Can you explain why it is you have never
    been seen by a dentist? **(probe)**

    ....

41. Do you think you will ever have to go to   Yes 1
    a dentist?   No 2
                                                  D.K. 3

42. Does the thought of wearing dentures   Yes 4
    bother you?   No 5
    If 'yes' or 'no'   D.K. 6
    Why do you think this?

    ....

43. (*a*) How well do you manage with the
        teeth you have?

        ....

    (*b*) Are you having any trouble with   Yes 7
        teeth or gums?   No 8
    If 'yes'   D.K. 9
    What sort of trouble?

    ....

    If 'no'
    If you had trouble with teeth or gums,
    what would you do about it?

    ....

F. NOW SOME GENERAL QUESTIONS

44. What do you look for when choosing a
    dentist?

    ....

45. Do you think what you do *now* to clean   Enough 1
    and take care of your teeth (dentures) is   Not enough 2
    enough or not enough?   D.K. 3
    If 'not enough'
    What else could you do?

    ....

46. Do you think what you did in the *past* to clean and take care of your teeth was enough or not enough?
    If 'not enough'
    What else could you have done?
    ....

Enough 4
Not enough 5
D.K. 6

47. (*a*) Would you rather go to a male or female dentist, or wouldn't it matter which?
    Probe answers except 'D.K.'
    Why do you say this?
    ....

Male 1
Female 2
Not matter............ 3
D.K. 4

   (*b*) Have you actually been treated by:

Male dentist only ... 5
Female dentist only 6
Both 7
D.K. 8

48. **Ask if only full-time employed (over 30 hour week) (do not ask if self-employed)**
    Does your employer usually allow time off to see a dentist?

Yes 1
No 2
D.K. 3

   If 'yes'
   Would you lose any money?

Yes 4
No 5
D.K. 6

49. If you went to the dentist today, how much treatment do you think you would need?

Now under
    treatment 1
None 2
Some 3
A lot 4
D.K. 5

50. (*a*) Do you think you have had about the same, more, or less trouble with your teeth than other people?
    (*b*) What has been the most troublesome thing that happened to your teeth?
    ....

About the same 1
More 2
Less 3
D.K. 4

51. (*a*) **Ask all except 'full denture'**

Does anyone in your family encour-   Yes 1
age you to visit the dentist?   No 2

                     D.n.a., no family

If 'yes'   F.D................... 3

Who does it?   ....   D.K. 4

(*b*) **Ask all**

Do you encourage anyone in your   Yes 5
family to visit the dentist?   No 6

                     D.n.a., no family,

                     F.D. 7

If 'yes'   D.K. 8

Whom ....

52. Perhaps you can tell me a little about your family?
I mean those members who live at this address.

                                Subject lives alone... 9

(Include children at boarding school or college—exclude lodgers)

Relation to subject (if son or daughter under 15 ask name)	Age (approx.)	Tooth status					Dentist				If child under 15 name of school
		Own teeth	No teeth yet	Partial denture	Full denture	D.K.	Goes to same dentist/practice	Goes to other dentist	Does not go/ Not for long time	D.K.	
		1	2	3	4	5	6	7	8	9	
		1	2	3	4	5	6	7	8	9	
		1	2	3	4	5	6	7	8	9	
		1	2	3	4	5	6	7	8	9	
		1	2	3	4	5	6	7	8	9	
		1	2	3	4	5	6	7	8	9	
		1	2	3	4	5	6	7	8	9	
		1	2	3	4	5	6	7	8	9	

G. FOR MOTHERS OF CHILDREN OVER 2 AND NOT YET 15

Now may I ask some questions about your children?

53. When do you think a child should first
be *examined* by a dentist? .... D.K.

54. Do you notice what state your children's Yes 1
teeth are in?   No 2
If 'yes'   D.K. 3
Just what do you notice?

....

		Child's name—look back to Qu. 52			
	Age:				
55.	What state do you think his/her teeth are in now?	Very good Good Fair Poor No teeth D.K.	Very good Good Fair Poor No teeth D.K.	Very good Good Fair Poor No teeth D.K.	Very good Good Fair Poor No teeth D.K.
56.	Would you like his/her teeth to be better?	Yes No D.K.	Yes No D.K.	Yes No D.K.	Yes No D.K.
57.	How much treatment do you think he/she needs now?	A lot Some Little None D.K.	A lot Some Little None D.K.	A lot Some Little None D.K.	A lot Some Little None D.K.
58.	Has he/she ever been *inspected* by a dentist? *If "yes"* At what age was the first time?	Yes No D.K. ... years D.K.	Yes No D.K. ... years D.K.	Yes No D.K. ... years D.K.	Yes No D.K. ... years D.K.
59.	*If "yes" to Qu. 58* When was the *last* visit to a dentist? (*probe carefully*)				
60.	When do you expect he/she will go *next*?				
61.	What does he/she think of going to the dentist? (*prompt*): Nervous of anything?				

ASK QU. 62 AND 63 IF HAS CHILDREN AT SCHOOL

What can you say about the school
dental service?

.... D.K.

Have any of your children been *treated* by   Yes 1
the school dentist?   No 2

    D.K. 3

If 'yes'   Very satisfied 4
(*a*) How satisfied have you been with   Fairly satisfied 5
treatment by the school dentist?   Not really satisfied... 6
If 'fairly' or 'not really satisfied'
Why is this?

....

(*b*) Do your children usually have their   School service 7
dental *treatment* through the school   Local dentist 8
service or the local dentist?   Both 9

    D.K. 0

64. Do you prefer your children to be treated   Male 1
by a male dentist, a female dentist, or   Female 2
doesn't it matter which?   Not matter 3

    D.K. 4

Probe answers except 'D.K.'
Why do you say this?

....

65. Have you ever had difficulty in getting   Yes 1
your children seen by a dentist?   No 2

    D.K. 3

If 'yes'
How was that?

....

66. (*a*) Do you think what your children do   Enough 1
to clean and take care of their teeth is   Not enough 2
enough or not enough?   D.K. 3
If 'not enough'
What else could they do?

....

(*b*) **If has child under 5:**
Do you clean his/her/their teeth?

Yes 4
No 5
D.K. 6

67. What do you think causes teeth to decay?
.... D.K.

68. (*a*) Are there any foods or drinks which your children have, that you know are good for their teeth?

Yes (specify) 1
No 2
D.K. 3

....

(*b*) Are there any foods or drinks which your children have, that you know are bad for their teeth?

Yes (specify) 4
No 5
D.K. 6

....

Did you have any special trouble with your teeth or gums during pregnancy?

Yes 7
No 8
D.K. 9

If 'yes'

69. (*a*) What was it? ....
(*b*) What did you do about it?
(If went to dentist—probe type of service) ....

Ask all:

70. (*a*) For the purpose of this survey would you be kind enough to let a dentist examine your teeth (dentures)? No treatment would be given, and we can arrange for him to call on you.

Yes 1
No 2
D.K. 3

(*b*) Do you think other members of your family living at this address would be willing to have their teeth examined?

Yes 4
No 5
D.K. 6

71. (*a*) Are there any changes you would like to see in the dental treatment services?

Yes (specify) 1
No 2
D.K. 3

....

(b) Do you have any particular com-   Yes (specify) 4
plaints about dental treatment?   No 5
....   D.K. 6

72. Is there anything else you would like to
say about your teeth or dentist?
....

PERSONAL DATA (SUBJECT)

Name ....   Sex M F   Age ...... years
Address ....   Marital status S M W D
....
Occupation ....   Employed: full time/part time/
self-employed.
Industry ....   (full time is over 30 hours/week)
(or work description)   If in full-time education
(specify): ....
If married woman—Husband's occupation: ....
(Main occupation if husband retired)
If widow—Husband's main occupation: ....
If subject retired—main occupation: ....
How long subject resident in this town (village): .... years
Previous place of residence: ....
Father's occupation—(When subject left school): ....
(If father then dead, last occupation)

THANK YOU VERY MUCH FOR ALL YOUR HELP—LEAVE LEAFLET

Appendix B. *Dental chart*

NAME	AGE	SEX	RECORD No.
		D	
		S	

DATE
TIME
EXR
REDR

DFA

H T

LAST VISIT:

DENTOFACIAL ANOM.

0	No. TRT REQD.
1	CLEFT PALATE
2	PROGNATHISM
3	DEEP OVERBITE
4	CROWDING
5	CLEFT LIP
6	RETROGNATHISM
7	OPEN BITE
8	SPACING
9	OTHER
10	

Denture	Age	Spare	I Comfort	II Fit	III Care	IV Condn.	V Aes.
Upper F P			A B C D	A B Aid	A' B	A B	A B
Lower F P			A B C D	A B Aid	A B	A B	A B

TOOTH	Rem.	M	O	D	L	B	Grade		DMF T	DMF S	deF	dF	G	P	C	B.P.
8								8								
7								7								
6								6								
5E								5E								
4D								4D								
3C								3C								
2B								2B								
1A								1A								
1A								1A								
2B								2B								
3C								3C								
4D								4D								
5E								5E								
6								6								
7								7								
8								8								

RIGHT — UPPER LEFT

8								8								
7								7								
6								6								
5E								5E								
4D								4D								
3C								3C								
2B								2B								
1A								1A								
1A								1A								
2B								2B								
3C								3C								
4D								4D								
5E								5E								
6								6								
7								7								
8								8								

LEFT — LOWER RIGHT

	Rem.	M	O	D	L	B	Totals						P	C	B.P.
Totals							32	160	20	20	20					

Appendix C. *Dental health of school children*

The programme for this survey did not provide specifically for any investigation of the dental health of children in school. A valuable source of information would, however, have been lost had no attempt been made to undertake such an investigation. Permission of the authorities in both towns was obtained to examine the children of four schools in Salisbury and three in Darlington. The types of schools and numbers of children were:

SALISBURY	Boys	Girls	Total
Infants	85	72	157
Infants	69	63	132
Secondary modern	0	364	364
Secondary modern	199	193	392
	353	692	1,045
DARLINGTON			
Infants	97	105	202
Secondary modern	178	0	178
Secondary modern	0	180	180
	275	285	560

These numbers gave reasonable coverage of the critical age-groups of 5–7 years, 11–14 years, and school-leavers. The examination technique used was the same as that used in the main survey: children from three of the schools being examined in the trailer and the remainder in the schools due to parking problems.

The results now presented are expressed in terms of dmf/DMF: the figure given being the number of teeth present in the average mouth. Teeth containing both decay and a restoration are classified as 'decayed' only. 'Missing' teeth do not include those shed naturally (deciduous) or those not yet erupted within reasonable eruption limits for the tooth in question. Only the major findings are presented in this Report; more detailed analysis will be the subject of a separate paper.

I. Infants

Age 5–7 years

This age-group covers the mature deciduous dentition, all teeth of which have been present in the mouth for about 2½ years at least; and includes the eruption of the first permanent tooth—the first molar. Permanent teeth are, however, not included in the following tables which are concerned solely with dmf values.

	5·0–5·5	5·6–5·11	6·0–6·5	6·6–6·11	Total 5·0–6·11
SALISBURY					
Average teeth per child					
Decayed (d)	2·9	3·4	3·7	3·5	3·4
Missing (m)	1·0	1·0	1·9	2·2	1·6
Filled (f)	0·6	0·9	0·7	0·8	0·7
Sound	15·2	14·1	11·7	10·4	12·8
Average total teeth present	19·7	19·4	18·0	16·9	18·5
Total children	53	48	65	60	226
DARLINGTON					
Average teeth per child					
Decayed (d)	3·7	3·9	3·6	4·7	4·0
Missing (m)	0·7	1·1	1·7	1·8	1·4
Filled (f)	0·1	0·0	0·0	0·1	0·0
Sound	15·5	14·6	13·2	10·8	13·2
Average total teeth present	20·0	19·6	18·5	17·4	18·6
Total children	31	35	38	48	152
Total dmf					
Salisbury	4·5	5·3	6·3	6·5	5·7
Darlington	4·5	5·0	5·3	6·6	5·4

There was no significant difference between the total dmf figures for the two towns; nor was there between the 'decayed' and 'missing' totals. There was, however, a significant difference between the 'filled' totals with a probability of 97·5 per cent. In other words, proportionally more teeth were filled in this age-range in Salisbury than in Darlington.

Within the age-range in both towns there was a tendency for the 'decayed' and 'missing' totals to increase slightly with age, while the 'filled' total remained constant. The number of teeth per child decreased with increasing age owing to the shedding of deciduous incisors as the permanent incisors erupted.

II. Secondary modern

Age 11–15½ years

The youngest children in this age-range have had at least some permanent teeth—the first molars—present in the mouth for 5 years, and have a complete permanent dentition except for the second molar, which will erupt at about 12 years and the third molar, due to erupt in the late teens or early 20s. Deciduous teeth are not included in the following tables.

	Age									Total
	11·0–11·5	11·6–11·11	12·0–12·5	12·6–12·11	13·0–13·5	13·6–13·11	14·0–14·5	14·6–14·11	15·0–15·5	11·0–15·5
SALISBURY										
Average teeth per child										
Decayed (D)	1·6	2·1	1·7	2·2	2·4	2·3	2·4	3·2	2·6	2·3
Missing (M)	0·3	0·7	0·8	1·6	1·6	1·1	2·0	2·2	1·9	1·4
Filled (F)	1·5	1·5	2·2	2·9	3·1	3·5	4·3	3·8	5·3	3·0
Sound	18·0	20·3	20·3	19·7	19·8	20·3	19·1	18·7	18·2	19·5
Average total teeth present	21·4	24·6	25·0	26·4	26·9	27·2	27·8	27·9	28·0	26·2
Total children	80	72	95	88	85	93	100	94	22	729
DARLINGTON										
Average teeth per child										
Decayed (D)	—	2·9	3·1	3·6	2·9	4·3	3·8	3·9	3·7	3·6
Missing (M)	—	0·7	1·0	1·2	1·4	1·8	2·7	2·2	3·0	1·9
Filled (F)	—	0·7	0·3	1·2	1·0	1·2	1·2	1·7	1·8	1·2
Sound	—	19·8	20·3	20·5	21·5	20·3	20·2	20·1	19·4	20·2
Average total teeth present	—	24·1	24·7	26·5	26·8	27·6	27·9	27·9	27·9	26·9
Total children	—	39	25	39	40	54	40	45	58	340
Total DMF										
Salisbury	3·4	4·3	4·7	6·7	7·1	6·9	8·7	9·2	9·8	6·7
Darlington	—	4·3	4·4	6·0	5·3	7·3	7·7	7·8	8·5	6·7

There was again no significant difference between the total DMF figures for the two towns, nor for the total 'missing' figures. Both the 'decayed' and 'filled' totals, however, differed significantly. This means that within this age-range Salisbury children had proportionally fewer decayed teeth and more filled teeth than Darlington. This reflects the adult dental-health picture already described and one factor must inevitably be the small number of dentists available in the school dental service in Darlington compared with Salisbury; even though the number in Salisbury was itself insufficient to deal with the total need.

As with deciduous teeth, there was a tendency within the age-range for total DMF to increase with age, and this was particularly marked in Salisbury, due almost entirely to an increase in the number of filled teeth. The lesser increase in Darlington was mainly due to contributions from both the 'missing' and 'filled' columns. In neither town was there a significant increase in the 'decayed' total, showing that within this age-range treatment was at least keeping pace with new decay in this particular sample. Obviously these figures do not represent the total school population of the two towns; this was not a random sample. They do, however, provide evidence of the over-all trends in each town. The fact that the later age-groups showed a higher total DMF in Salisbury than in Darlington does not necessarily indicate a higher decay rate in Salisbury. The higher proportion of teeth filled in Salisbury included restoration of some teeth whose decay was unregistered by our examination methods. The use of bite-wing radiographs, for example, would have increased proportionally the 'decayed' totals at the expense of the 'sound' totals—a difference probably sufficient to account for the total DMF differences in the later age-groups.

Appendix D. *Oral health grading*

In order to produce a reasonably accurate picture of the dental health of a community, it is necessary to consider not only the incidence of each type of oral disease—dental decay, periodontal disease; but also the total effect of all disease processes acting in the mouth. To use an obvious example, it is not uncommon for gross periodontal disease to flourish in a decay-free mouth. Looked at in terms of dental decay alone, this is a healthy mouth—yet without treatment of the perio-dontal condition these same healthy teeth are doomed to early loss. Similarly, grossly decayed teeth may exist in a healthy periodontium, especially in young people. Therefore, to quote a figure of so many people with a sound dentition in the broad context of oral health is misleading, if not quite useless. What is required is an index of oral health which will take into account the condition of all oral tissues. The compilation of such an index, however, creates many problems and the attempt now to be described is merely one step towards a satisfactory solution. Because of its limitations, this attempt is better described as an oral health grading rather than an oral health index.

General oral health may be considered under three major headings: dental, periodontal, and prosthetic. It could be argued that an ortho-dontic heading should be included, but for practical reasons this would tend to over-complicate a system which must of necessity be kept as simple as accuracy will permit. In practice nothing is lost by the omission of orthodontic information. It is now necessary to provide a system of grades for each of these three main divisions and three such grades, corresponding to 'good', 'fair', and 'poor' are considered to be adequate. More than three gradings leads to confusion in definition and interpretation, and less than three to lack of adequate information. An exception may be made in the prosthetic division, where only two grades are required—'satisfactory' and 'unsatisfactory'—since a denture either fits or it does not; it is required or it is not required. Here, then, is the foundation for an oral health grading, whereby a six-digit code will give a measure of the oral health of any subject. The three divisions are referred to by letter, i.e. A (dental), B (periodontal), and C (prosthetic) and the three grades by figures—1, 2, and 3; or in the case of the prosthetic division 1 and 3. Thus an entirely healthy mouth would be classified as A1B1C1 while severe dental decay in an otherwise healthy mouth would result in a classification of A3B1C1.

When it comes to defining the grades in each division, extracted teeth present something of a problem. A missing tooth, if it leaves a gap in the dental arch, represents a partial but irreversible failure to maintain an ideal standard of oral health. The gap may be filled by a prosthesis, but like any other artificial substitute this is at best a second-rate alternative, with considerable limitations. A successful restoration, on the other hand, represents a complete return of a tooth to its fully functional place in the dental arch—with some reservations in the case of silicate restorations where some functional efficiency has to be sacrificed for aesthetic appearance. Logically, therefore, missing teeth must receive a lower grading than even heavily decayed teeth, since the latter may be capable of complete restoration while the former can only be replaced by a prosthesis. Similarly a non-existent periodontium can hardly be graded higher than even a grossly diseased periodontium which is nevertheless still performing its proper function of supporting the teeth.

Two points of interpretation arise from this. Firstly, oral health cannot be related entirely to treatment needs since, for example, an A3 grading may refer to loss of all or nearly all teeth with no further treatment requirements or it may refer to gross decay in all teeth which will require lengthy treatment. In other words the grading will provide a measure of oral neglect rather than oral needs. Secondly, and arising from this, it is not possible to differentiate between denture wearers and others. A3B3C1 could apply equally to a full denture wearer with satisfactory dentures and someone with all their natural teeth but all grossly decayed and with a heavily diseased periodontium. This problem may be overcome to some extent by dividing the A3B3C1 and A3B3C3 groups into full denture wearers and others. One alternative would have been to introduce four grades into the prosthetic division; two dealing with the need for dentures and two dealing with the adequacy of existing dentures. However, this tended to cause more complications than its use justified.

Following now are the definitions used for the various grades. These definitions must inevitably be capable of fairly liberal interpretation, depending on subject age and similar relevant factors; decay, for example, in a young person is less desirable than decay in an older person and likely to be more serious, from an oral health viewpoint.

Dental

*A*I. At least two molar teeth must be present in each quadrant, and the dental arch must be continuous, with no gaps. All teeth must be free from decay, although one minimal cavity may be present in the whole mouth. Restorations may be unlimited, providing that they are satisfactory. The presence of dentures or bridges automatically rules out an AI classification, since they indicate a break in the continuity of the dental arch.

*A*2. This grade includes all cases not qualifying as AI or A3.

*A*3. Normally more than half the teeth are missing, although in an older person 15 sound teeth present could qualify for an A2 grading. Similarly a young person with 20 badly decayed teeth present would be graded A3.

As a general rule, AI grades require no treatment and have sound teeth; A2 either need treatment to bring them to a complete state of dental fitness or else have lost part of their natural dentition and require treatment to save permanently the remainder; and A3 have either completely lost their natural dentition or else have some part remaining which probably cannot be permanently saved by restorative means. Thus some A2s could become AI after treatment, but hardly any A3s could become A2, and none could become AI.

Periodontal

*B*I. No pathological gingival pocketing, inflammation must be restricted to no more than 2 teeth and only isolated spots of calculus are permitted except in the lower anterior region where all four incisors may show limited amounts. At least two-thirds of the normal periodontium must be present—i.e. at least 20 teeth must be present.

*B*2. This grade includes all cases not qualifying as BI or B3.

*B*3. Pathological pocketing in excess of 3 mm. around more than 2 teeth, and gross general calculus coupled with gross chronic inflammation. In young people less calculus and inflammation would still qualify for a B3 grading. Less than one-third of the periodontium remaining (less than 9 teeth present) would also earn a B3 grading.

As a general rule B1 grades require no treatment other than a routine scale and polish, while B2 grades require more elaborate periodontal treatment and even then, as a result of tooth loss, may not qualify for a B1 grading. B3 grades will normally, except in cases of extensive tooth loss require prolonged periodontal treatment including gingivectomy, and even then the prognosis would probably be poor if not hopeless.

Prosthetic

C1. *Either* no dentures or bridges are worn or required, *or* dentures and/or bridges are worn and are functioning satisfactorily.

C3. *Either* no dentures or bridges are worn but are required, *or* dentures and/or bridges are worn and need repair or replacement.

A bridge or denture is considered to be necessary if a gap of more than one unit exists in either arch or if more than one molar is missing in any quadrant.

'C' gradings may be related directly to treatment, since in C1 cases treatment is not required and in C3 cases prosthetic treatment is necessary.

If any population is graded according to this classification, all subjects may be placed in 1 of 15 categories or classes (not 18, because by definition no-one can be classified A1B1C3, A1B2C3, or A1B3C3). If the A3B3C1 and A3B3C3 classes are subdivided into denture and non-denture wearers this raises the number of classes to 17. It would now be useful to list these 17 classes in a descending order of oral health but again complications arise. The extreme ends of the scale present no problem—at the top there is A1B1C1 and at the bottom A3B3C3, with or without dentures. Between these limits, however, the order must to a great extent be arbitrary, and liable to dispute. Is periodontal health more important than dental health? Should A2C1B1 be rated higher than A1B2C1? In practice the problem is simplified by the fact that most people in a cross-sectional adult population tend to fall mainly into only 5 or 6 of the 17 classes. These, in order of 'popularity' are:

1. A3B3C3—full denture wearers
2. A3B3C1—full denture wearers
3. A3B3C3—non-full denture wearers
4. A2B1C1
5. A2B2C1
6. A2B3C3
7. A1B1C1—young age-groups only

These six categories alone seem to account for 75 per cent of the average population. At the other end of the scale five classes are hardly used. These are:

1. A3B1C1	4. A1B3C1
2. A1B2C1	5. A3B1C3
3. A3B2C1	

These account for 5 per cent or less of the average total population. If these last 5 classes are ignored, it would seem reasonable to 'score' the remaining 12 classes by adding together the A and B grades and to this total adding one for a C3 grading and subtracting one for a C1 grading. This would give an order as follows:

Class	Score	Class	Score
A1B1C1	1	A2B2C3	5
A2B1C1	2	A3B3C1 (NFD)	5
A2B2C1	3	A3B2C3	6
A2B1C3	4	A2B3C3	6
A2B3C1	4	A3B3C3 (NFD)	7

Class	
A3B3C1 (FD)	} unscored
A3B3C3 (FD)	

The only illogicality in this order would appear to be the placing of A3B3C1 above A3B2C3, and even this may be merely a matter of opinion.

The individual may, therefore, be given an oral health score of between 1 and 7 which should quite accurately reflect the oral health state, although with the exception of the extreme scores of 1 and 7 it would give little indication of treatment needs.

The results of our investigations are now presented to illustrate this method of oral health grading.

	Score (percentage totals)							FD satisfactory	FD unsatisfactory
	1	2	3	4	5	6	7		
SALISBURY									
Males	2	8	9	8	5	11	14	8	34
Females	5	13	6	6	8	11	10	11	30
DARLINGTON									
Males	2	5	8	6	8	10	10	22	26
Females	6	4	5	7	9	6	9	26	26

These results show an over-all similarity between the two towns and between the two sexes in each town. There was, however, a tendency for oral health to be better in Salisbury than in Darlington, and in both towns better in women than in men. A more realistic assessment may be made if the full denture wearers are ignored; the table then becomes:

	1	2	3	4	5	6	7
SALISBURY							
Males	3	14	15	15	9	19	25
Females	9	22	10	10	13	19	18
DARLINGTON							
Males	4	10	17	13	16	19	20
Females	13	9	12	16	18	13	19
Salisbury total	6	18	12	12	11	19	21
Darlington total	8	10	15	15	17	16	20

Age distribution

Oral health grading

Age	Score (percentages)							FD satisfactory	FD unsatisfactory
	1	2	3	4	5	6	7		
SALISBURY									
21–5	11	38	17	8	6	8	5	0	8
26–30	13	17	22	12	18	13	4	0	0
31–5	3	17	9	20	6	11	23	3	9
36–40	0	11	15	8	8	18	16	8	16
41–5	7	10	9	9	7	9	16	7	26
46–50	3	6	0	6	6	17	14	11	37
51–5	0	0	0	9	5	26	17	13	30
56–60	0	0	0	0	0	8	12	12	68
61–5	0	0	0	0	6	3	7	20	63
66–70	0	0	0	0	8	0	8	25	58
Over 70	0	0	0	0	4	0	8	19	69
DARLINGTON									
21–5	15	26	18	15	23	3	0	0	0
26–30	17	8	22	13	14	13	8	0	5
31–5	6	11	17	18	12	17	6	11	3
36–40	8	6	11	14	20	6	11	11	14
41–5	0	5	5	8	8	8	18	24	24
46–50	0	0	4	6	4	13	9	30	34
51–5	0	0	0	2	2	10	8	46	32
56–60	0	0	0	0	3	6	8	33	50
61–5	0	0	0	4	8	0	14	39	36
66–70	0	0	5	0	0	9	18	36	32
Over 70	0	0	0	0	3	0	9	33	55

Omitting full denture wearers

Oral health grading

Age	Score (percentages)						
	1	2	3	4	5	6	7
SALISBURY							
21–5	12	41	18	9	6	9	6
26–30	13	17	22	12	18	13	4
31–5	3	19	10	23	6	13	26
36–40	0	14	21	10	10	24	21
41–5	10	14	14	14	10	14	24
46–50	5	11	0	11	11	33	28
51–5	0	0	0	15	8	46	31
56–60	0	0	0	0	0	40	60
61–5	0	0	0	0	40	20	40
66–70	0	0	0	0	50	0	50
Over 70	0	0	0	0	33	0	67
DARLINGTON							
21–5	15	26	18	15	23	3	0
26–30	18	8	23	14	15	14	8
31–5	7	13	19	20	14	19	7
36–40	11	8	14	18	26	8	14
41–5	0	9	9	15	15	15	36
46–50	0	0	11	17	11	36	25
51–5	0	0	0	9	9	45	36
56–60	0	0	0	0	18	35	77
61–5	0	0	0	15	31	0	55
66–70	0	0	16	0	0	28	56
Over 70	0	0	0	0	25	0	75